MOLECULAR EVOLUTIONARY MODELS IN DRUG DISCOVERY

MOLECULAR EVOLUTIONARY MODELS IN DRUG DISCOVERY

JUAN BUENO, MD, MSc
Research Center of Bioprospecting and Biotechnology for Biodiversity Foundation (BIOLABB), Colombia

ELSEVIER
ACADEMIC PRESS
An imprint of Elsevier

Academic Press is an imprint of Elsevier
125 London Wall, London EC2Y 5AS, United Kingdom
525 B Street, Suite 1650, San Diego, CA 92101, United States
50 Hampshire Street, 5th Floor, Cambridge, MA 02139, United States
The Boulevard, Langford Lane, Kidlington, Oxford OX5 1GB, United Kingdom

Library of Congress Cataloging-in-Publication Data
A catalog record for this book is available from the Library of Congress

British Library Cataloguing-in-Publication Data
A catalogue record for this book is available from the British Library

ISBN 978-0-12-817613-9

For information on all Academic Press publications
visit our website at https://www.elsevier.com/books-and-journals

Publisher: Andre Wolff
Acquisition Editor: Erin Hill-Parks
Editorial Project Manager: Samantha Allard
Production Project Manager: Maria Bernard
Designer: Mark Rogers

Typeset by SPi Global, India

Dedication

To Martha Ritoré who patiently helped me in the evolution that led me to this book

To my father who patiently waited for me while I was thinking about the book

Contents

Preface

Biology on the planet has evolved from chance and necessity, just as Jacques Monod (1910–76) theorized. In this order of ideas, chance is represented by environmental challenges that exert stress on the biological system so that it initiates phenotypic adaptations, which when made functional become heritable and are transmitted to the following generations. Necessity is represented in the search of the living being to continue to function by using nutrients for energy, reproducing, and defending its space. To achieve functionality by virtue of the game of chance and the need that has shaped our biosphere, biological systems enter into communication and association so that in symbiosis they acquire fitness and the ability to transcend from an RNA world to an open biological system in constant exchange. And in this way, by virtue of association, communication, and mutualism, the biological entity holobiont conformed by a host and its symbionts emerges as an evolutionary model that allows biological systems to acquire autopoiesis (produce themselves) and autocatakinetics (organize themselves to themselves) with the consequent ability to share the entropy and configure metabolic networks for this purpose. On the other hand, the holobiont communicates with other holobionts in its ecosystem, configuring a network known as the meta-holobiont. This meta-holobiont is a superorganism in its communication process and acquires molecular evolution able to give greater capacity of fitness to the biological system and consequently of adaptation. Thus by assuming the human being as a holobiont, a biological system in constant ecoevolution and search for adaptation, it is possible to achieve another vision of medicine based on the complex systems with which a functional model can be developed to design new symbiotic medications. This symbiotic therapy is defined as reestablishment of ecosystemic equilibrium for treatment of the human holobiont. This reestablishment seeks to avoid tissue invasion and uncontrolled growth to achieve a correct thermodynamic homeostasis. This approach is also based on the quaternity of the exchange in an open biological system that consists of:

1. interaction
2. communication
3. transformation
4. evolution

Likewise, the characteristics of a symbiotic medication administered alone or in synergistic formulation are:

1. Allows and regulates phenotypic adaptations within the holobiont
2. Restores metabolic networks that allow energy exchange within the holobiont
3. Helps maintain and restore the thermodynamic equilibrium in the sharing of entropy
4. Maintains mutualistic interactions between the host and its symbionts
5. Induces proliferation of beneficial microbial species for the microbiome
6. Restores the homeosis between microbiome and host
7. Controls pathogenic microorganisms mediated by stimulation of probiotic microbial consortia
8. Does not present antimicrobial activity on the microbiome
9. Does not present toxicity against the symbiotic holobiont as a whole

Therefore in the context of personalized medicine, the criterion of the 4Ps (predictive, preventive, participatory, and personalized) should include a new factor that represents the evolution of the biological system, which we call the fifth P, pliability. We include pliability in order to complete the missing information as well as its correlations for the design and development of pharmacological innovations.

The main objective of this book is to integrate evolution as a biological phenomenon that has shaped the biosphere to the search and development of therapeutic innovations for use in medicine, agriculture, and industry. But for this we must connect the holobiont and its symbionts as the functional biological unit in association and communication that has emerged as a strategy to reach thermodynamic equilibrium and to that extent continue the metabolic flow of energy in the system.

Juan Bueno
Bogotá, Colombia

CHAPTER 1

Molecular evolution: The origins of interaction

It was in these circumstances... in which he analyzed Don Quixote's dilemma of whether to follow the path of arms (praxis, action) or the path of letters (poiesis, creation, production), I understood for the first time the power of the word "poiesis" and invented the word that we needed: autopoiesis. This was a word without a history, a word that could directly mean what takes place in the dynamics of the autonomy proper to living systems.

Humberto Maturana (1928–) and Francisco Varela (1946–2001)

Only love expands intelligence. To live in love is to accept the other and the conditions of his existence as a source of richness, not as opposition, restriction or limitation.

Humberto Maturana (1928–)

1.1 Introduction

The study of the evolution of biological molecules itself is nothing other than the evaluation of quasicrystals or aperiodic crystals (Maciá, 2005). This aperiodic order (orderly but without symmetry) has been the key to diversity and evolution since the appearance of the first molecules that had the capacity to self-replicate and with the ability to obtain memory patterns for future living systems (Jacobs & Frenkel, 2016; Zenil, 2013). Thus, prebiotic chemistry, like all forms, has physical laws that determine it, such as the state of the matter (Cleaves, 2018; Spitzer, Pielak, & Poolman, 2015), but the set of these laws that allow the origin of life from the interaction of molecules requires the nonlinearity of the dynamic process as well as the chaos that chance induces (Detrain & Deneubourg, 2006; Longo, Montévil, & Kauffman, 2012; Strogatz, 2018). That is why starting from molecular evolution as a primordial that is nourished by the interaction and communication between biological systems and their environment is probably the gateway

Molecular Evolutionary Models in Drug Discovery
https://doi.org/10.1016/B978-0-12-817613-9.00001-8

to a set of foundations that will regulate a future series of biotechnological applications (Barge et al., 2017; Wagner & Rosen, 2014). In this way, the game of biological macromolecules is established through interaction and communication that ultimately achieves the storage of useful information (Massey & Mishra, 2018).

This information on complex biological systems will determine the appearance of replicators that will initiate adaptive mutation processes when they come into contact with the environment and its changes (Ma'ayan, 2017; Melkikh, 2014). This is how molecular evolution will modulate phenotypic changes in different species as a means to achieve this adaptation (Chevin & Beckerman, 2012; Harms & Thornton, 2013). These challenges are also used as a means of molecular innovation that increases chemical diversity and resilience capacity to assume the external pressure that will allow evolutionary success (López-Maury, Marguerat, & Bähler, 2008). Finally, the macromolecules were diversified into the correspondence between the information represented by the genome and the functionality represented by the genotype both in their constant exchange of the environment (Sharov, 2014). Additionally, the thermodynamic flow that establishes the self-sustainability of the molecular evolution process must be taken into account to elucidate fluxomics in the production of metabolites, both primary and secondary (Kleidon, Malhi, & Cox, 2010). This is how the methods of evolutionary engineering appear as a consilient platform to develop chemical diversity of the capacity to use the adaptive potential for the species (Arnold, 2015; Shepelin, Hansen, Lennen, Luo, & Herrgård, 2018); all this comes from the study of social interactions between living organisms, which evolved from the exercise in communication as a means of survival (Flemming et al., 2016). The objective of this chapter will be to analyze the physical, chemical, and biological systems that make up the molecular interaction and that constitute a factor of evolution whose foundations will be applied in evolutionary engineering models.

1.2 Aperiodic crystals and biological molecules

The organization of complex biological systems is bound to the laws of physics, in particular to quantum mechanics, which establishes the capacity for innovation and evolution of species in thermodynamic flows (Katsnelson, Wolf, & Koonin, 2018). In this way, the primordial/prebiotic soup composed of aperiodic crystals (conformed molecules in a nonperiodic ordered structure) capable of self-replicating were fundamental for the appearance

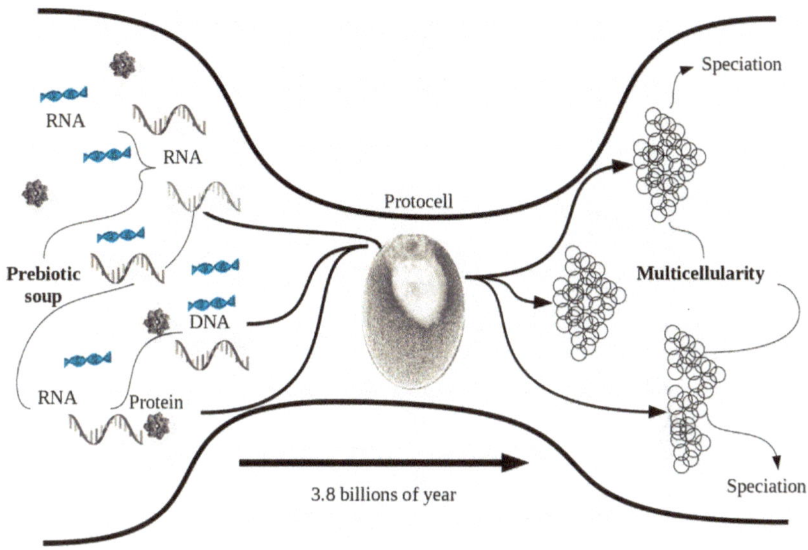

Fig. 1 Evolution of life from prebiotic soup until the protocell origin and multicellular organization.

of the first symbiotic cell or protobiont that came into interaction (Fig. 1) (Longo, Montévil, Sonnenschein, & Soto, 2015). Also, the physical and chemical properties of these molecules predispose to their micro-scale organization what preprogrammed their use in different cellular functions in the guise of an evolutionary geometry that lost periodicity or symmetry when they are represented in a three-dimensional space like regular crystals (Fig. 2) (Jorgenson, Mohammed, Agrawal, & Schulman, 2017; Murr, 2015). Likewise, these structures capable of carrying information are the link between an abiotic world and the emergence of life (Varn & Crutchfield, 2016; Wills, 2016). Equally, it is very important to take into account the emergence of autocatalytic sets, in which the symbiotic protobiont emerges from a group of molecules that formed a cooperative network that self-replicated together (Walker, 2017). Additionally, the autocatalytic network will be established as it acquires a state of homeostatic organization that allows it to configure a complex biosystem (Eskov, Filatova, Eskov, & Gavrilenko, 2017); in other words, it becomes self-sustaining and by compartmentalizing, it acquires the characteristics of a protocell (Hordijk, Naylor, Krasnogor, & Fellermann, 2018). Consequently, in the present living cells, the fact of being a nonperiodic molecular structure allows the interaction and the union of lengths, sizes, and forms into irregular configuration, as it is in those that the biological processes are developed (Polesskaya et al., 2018).

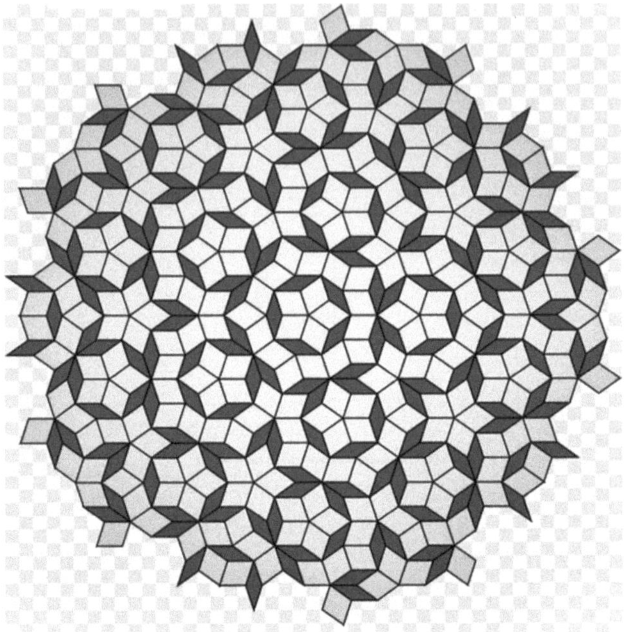

Fig. 2 Aperiodic structure of quasicrystal based on a Penrose tiling.

It is also important to note that this prebiotic chemistry that subsequently accumulated in vesicles required three fundamental processes: integration with the vesicle to prevent its degradation, stabilization of the structure of the vesicle in a symbiotic model, and finally, the development of a function in the role as protocell, all as part of the same life that is governed by physical-chemical laws (Mayer, Schreiber, & Dávila, 2015, 2017). In order for these ideas to acquire their function, the protocell established a metabolic network perpetuated in genetic information consigned to aperiodic crystal structures (De Tiège, 2017). Thus, from this abiotic world, through interaction, the different hierarchies of biological systems were reached, from a molecular level to a population level (Tëmkin & Eldredge, 2015). In this way, a crucial factor of the interactions within the protocols is the establishment of hyper cycles, in which self-replicating molecules such as RNA and DNA constitute cyclic connections that are autocatalytic (Sardanyés, Lázaro, Guillamon, & Fontich, 2017). It is in these hyper cycles where the interactions between the proteins reached self-sustaining processes of replication and communication allowed the origin of life (Andras & Andras, 2005); everything from a primordial soup of aperiodic crystals. But although Erwin Scrödinger suggested that these crystals would have the capacity to carry information (in his words, a "Morse code") that leads to survival through communication (Zwart, 2018), it is necessary to discuss a little more as each protocol entered into symbiosis with its neighbors.

1.3 Cell-to-cell communication

Our microbial ancestors developed communication systems initially to perceive and control low population density of different conditions of environmental nutrients; the best known is called quorum sensing, which is an early-onset mechanism in bacteria (Lerat & Moran, 2004; Schluter, Schoech, Foster, & Mitri, 2016). The system of quorum sensing regulates the cooperation of microbial cells in response to external pH and stress as factors, inducing different functions such as replication, gene exchange, and formation of biofilm associations (Moreno-Gámez et al., 2017). Likewise, as the system becomes redundant due to the development of several molecular signaling pathways, it acquires complexity, forming information networks within cell communities (Even-Tov et al., 2016). Finally, these forms of communication determined the processes that led to endosymbiotic relationships between α-proteobacteria and the archaean host, which led to the appearance of mitochondria as a metabolic organelle (Chandel, 2015). This fusion, which was derived from the role of the activation of quorum sensing during the increase in the population density and the decrease of nutrients, was able to promote survival and adaptation during shortage of energy resources (Picard & Burelle, 2012). For that reason, the evolutionary adaptations of the signaling system focus on the intracellular distribution of carbon and energy resources (Wu et al., 2016). Additionally, as these self-inductors produced in the quorum sensing achieved the adaptation for survival, they also had a primordial role in the establishment of a symbiotic network of interaction with other microorganisms in constant evolution of the constitution of structured communities with ecosystem functions as the form of a biofilm (Hansen, Rainey, Haagensen, & Molin, 2007). This formation favored the primordial microorganisms to achieve an adaptive diversification into the ecosystem niche that confers cooperation and exchange with information on different microbial populations (Steenackers, Parijs, Foster, & Vanderleyden, 2016).

1.4 Biofilm as an evolutionary niche

In microbial ecology, the adaptation and survival of different species was a fundamental factor of establishing the evolutionary process that developed terrestrial biodiversity (Van Der Heijden, Bardgett, & Van Straalen, 2008), also constituting a terrestrial microbiome in constant exchange (Fröhlich-Nowoisky et al., 2016). In this way, microorganisms from the origin of life have established themselves as the greatest promoters of biodiversity, due to the ability to perform symbiosis with other organisms in a constant exchange of information within a hologenome that groups the coded information of both the host and the microbiota with which it is in contact (Rosenberg & Zilber-Rosenberg, 2018; Zilber-Rosenberg & Rosenberg, 2008). In this conformation of the symbiotic holobionts (microbial communities and their host both plant and animal), the biofilm has played a fundamental role in the establishment of a microbial ecosystem that can interact as a whole with its symbiont (Doolittle & Booth, 2017). This is how, when conceiving modern living beings as multi organismal entities, it is possible to determine the influence of microorganisms on the physiology, metabolism and molecular signaling inside the host (Douglas, 2018). In addition, Bordenstein and Theis (2015) had postulated the basic principles of holobionts and hologenomes that should be taken into consideration when approaching these complex systems as a driver of molecular evolution, such as:

1. Holobionts and hologenomes are complex biological systems.
2. Holobionts and hologenomes should not be considered an organ system, as well as superorganisms or metagenomes.
3. The hologenome should be studied as a genetic system itself.
4. The notion of the hologenome reinforces and employs elements of the Lamarckian evolutionary model.
5. Changes in the hologenome are subject to mutation mechanisms
6. The hologenomic evolution should be understood in terms that equate a gene within the nuclear genome with the microorganism within the microbiome.
7. The abstraction of the hologenome is adapted to the fundamentals of genetics, as well as to the group selection theory.
8. The hologenome is determined by the concepts of selection as well as neutrality.
9. Hologenomic speciation integrates the concepts of genetics and symbiosis.
10. Holobionts and hologenomes do not alter the fundamentals of evolutionary biology, they reinforce them.

Likewise, this holobiont through the symbiotic interactions that are established within sociomicrobiological formations such as biofilms acquires the ability to evolve in a phenotypic manner, which allows it to persist in different environmental conditions (Haag, 2018). This gives value of co-operative processes and to the exchange as a generator of diversity within the present biological system (Muraille, 2018), finally resulting in biological innovation in conjunction with the morphological diversity that characterizes species with a high level of adaptation (Nguyen et al., 2016). These innovations are crucial moments in the origin of life when defining the appearance of functions that optimize interaction and communication within an ecosystem (Hochberg, Marquet, Boyd, & Wagner, 2017).

It is also important to consider the role of the biofilm within the notion of developmental evolutionary biology (evo-devo), where epigenetic regulations can transform the architecture of microbial formation (Brockman et al., 2018; Love, 2015). In this aspect it is important to note that, although some authors do not consider the biofilm as a biological individual (Clarke, 2016), the fact of constituting itself as an ecosystem that groups microbial communities makes it a biological entity to be studied as a whole. Important evidence in this regard is the phenotypic heterogeneity present in the bacteria that results in the appearance of several subpopulations that adapt to different environmental changes without altering the DNA sequence (Casadesús & Low, 2013). Therefore, it is tempting to consider the biofilm as an ancient multicellular structure of a metabolism and organic structure that is part of an epiphenomenon regulated by its interaction with the environment and its signaling molecules present in the quorum sensing system (Torday & Miller, 2016). In this sense, it has been possible to determine the presence of multicellular aggregates inside the biofilms, which reinforces the concept that the natural form of the bacteria is living within these microbial formations and not in an isolated way (Kragh et al., 2016). Finally, this acquires importance in the sense that the multicellularity becomes a great biological innovation where the molecular evolution goes from being a microscopic aspect to beginning to constitute itself in a macroscopic organization (Lyons & Kolter, 2015).

1.5 The rise of macroscopic symbiotic holobionts

The process of symbiogenesis results from the constant interaction of organisms in the conformation of a holobiont (Guerrero, Margulis, & Berlanga, 2013). This translates into a molecular evolution of speciation that is characterized by being homeostatic and autopoietic—that is, an organism in communication with a self-sustaining metabolic equilibrium (O'Malley, 2017); communication that seeks the adaptation of living systems and that led protobionts to be holobionts (De Loof, 2017). But for this process, it is necessary to achieve a vectorial biochemistry inside the cell with which it is possible to start a metabolution platform (Spitzer & Poolman, 2009). This is how it has been shown that changes in metabolic pathways can lead to an improvement in the adaptive behavior of organisms, which leads to an increase in their evolutionary capacities (Egbert, Barandiaran, & Di Paolo, 2011). Additionally, living organisms are not unique individuals in isolation; they constitute a great network of metabolites in constant interaction, communication, mutation, and evolution that constitute the symbiotic holobiont (Gilbert, Sapp, & Tauber, 2012). Thus we see that the multicellular organism in interaction becomes a metaorganism (Fig. 3), which acquires a relation of synergistic interdependence with its symbionts (Bang et al., 2018).

The notion of metaorganisms introduces us to a primordial pattern of molecular evolution, which is co-evolution, in which genomes, phenotypes, and ecosystems are connected, modeling the evolutionary process (Bosch & McFall-Ngai, 2011). Co-evolution as an integrating concept gives us the possibility of explaining the processes that have shaped life on earth through molecularly mediated interaction, as well as teaching us its role as a driver of diversity (Carmona, Fitzpatrick, & Johnson, 2015). The ultimate goal of this co-evolutionary process is to achieve greater complexity of the systems; therefore, the level of evolution is measured in degree of complexity, which translates into greater capacity for interaction and communication (Ekstig, 2015; Futuyma & Agrawal, 2009). Also these complex systems (Fig. 4) must have

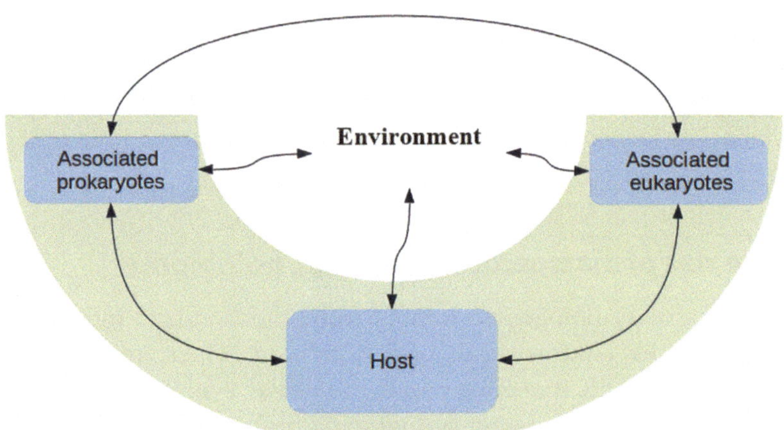

Fig. 3 Metaorganism structure conformed by the host and their associations with prokaryotes, eukaryotes, and environment.

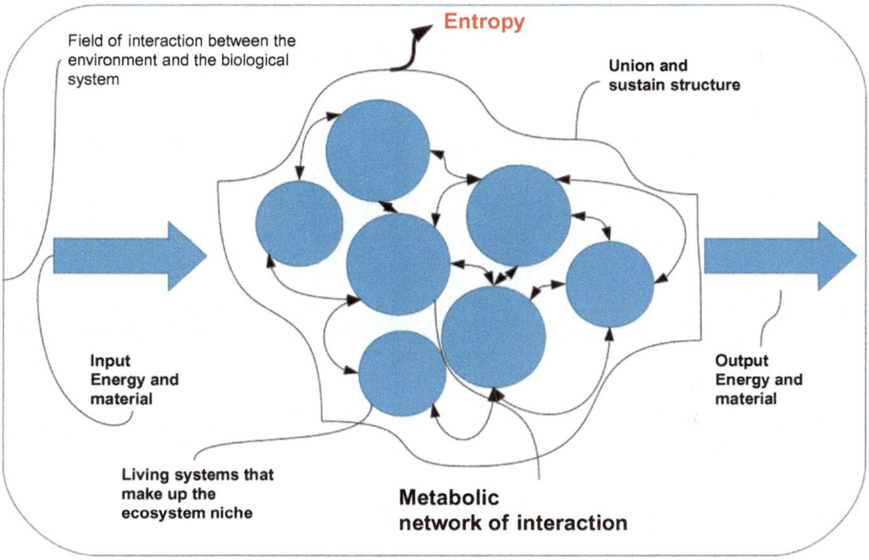

Fig. 4 Configuration of a complex biological system and its symbiotic interactions.

two components defined as microstate and macrostate, where both the interactions to form the macrostate and the transformations of the interactions between the elements of the microstate are established, this is achieved through a dynamic influence and exchange (Holovatch, Kenna, & Thurner, 2017). This guarantees the thermodynamic equilibrium and the energy flow inside the system as well as determining its structure and shape; this under a signaling system with two characteristics: a detectable amount of transmitted energy and a time of action (Fenzl, 2018). Additionally, life also depends on the flow of information to reproduce, look for food, protection, and act in conjunction with the biological network to face environmental changes (Tkačik & Bialek, 2016).

On the other hand, when shaping the biological networks and their energy flow, the different complex mixtures of molecules acquire their function by virtue of the interactions that they establish. The study of these systems must be done as a whole group (Sun & Wu, 2015), and it is in these signaling cascades that the systems become autocatalytic under the modulation of reversible covalent reactions in the integration of multiple equilibrium (Ren & You, 2015). For this reason, it is the living systems that work in nonequilibrium conditions that keep the gradients and the transport of molecules active, with the consequent continuous flow of functional processes (Grzybowski & Huck, 2016). This is why it is in these factors of

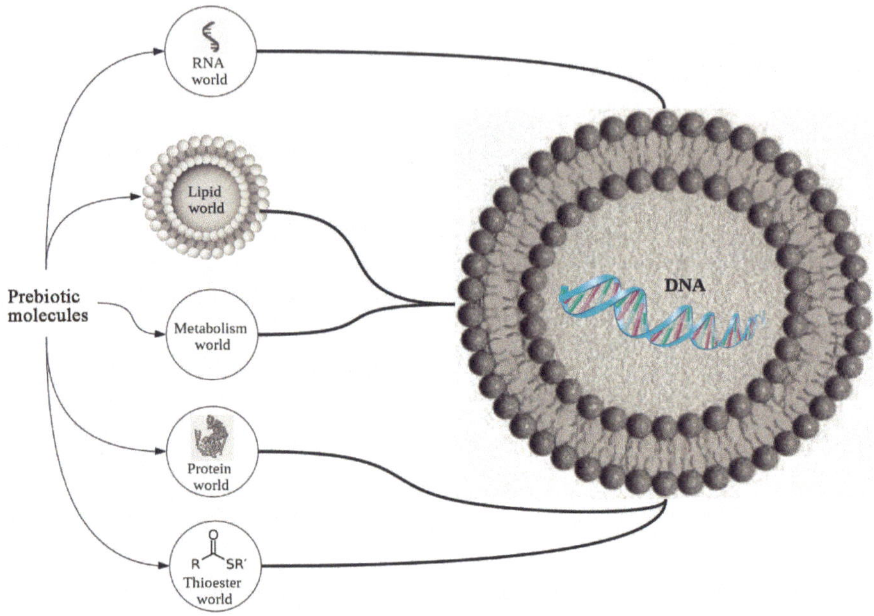

Fig. 5 Prebiotic worlds—supramolecular entities that in homogeneous union of heterogeneous compounds configure the chemical bases of the origin of life as a self-replicating and self-sustaining entity.

supramolecular chemistry that we have to look for the systems that make up life as a holistic interaction of elements (Sevim et al., 2018). Likewise, this union of supramolecular entities constituted in a homogeneous class of heterogeneity (proteins, nucleic acids, polysaccharides, lipid bilayers) (Fig. 5) reached their highest degree of complexity in favor of interaction, communication, and adaptation until it became a biological macrostate (Krishnamurthy, 2017).

1.6 Secondary metabolism: Innovations for survival

The study of secondary metabolism by virtue of co-evolution has focused on being a metadiscipline that unites natural biomedical agents, the functional properties of biomolecules, as well as their interactions (Allard et al., 2018). In this sense, the evolution of chemical diversity is linked to biomolecular activity that favors the organism capable of developing the appropriate metabolic pathways that reduce the energy cost of producing secondary metabolites (Firn & Jones, 2000; Tianero et al., 2016). For this reason, the production of this type of compound, which is foreign to the functions of growth, reproduction, and development of the biological system, is part of a special role in increasing the competitive capabilities of the organisms that synthesize them (Jenke-Kodama, Müller, & Dittmann, 2008). Then, it is determined that the ecological and physiological function of these compounds is no other than to regulate the interaction between the symbiotic holobionts within the metaorganisms (Giordano et al., 2015). This produces an ecological niche, coming from the mutual adaptation resulting from the constant interaction and the mutual construction of structures for the development (Chiu & Gilbert, 2015). In addition, these interaction networks modulated the appearance of biosynthetic gene clusters (BGCs) as a source of diversity and chemical innovation (Bapteste & Huneman, 2018). This has been demonstrated in the ability of BGCs to evolve into new functionalities using redundancies in genetic information that allow progress in the direction of other functions, target based, but without losing the original functions (Hoogendoorn et al., 2018).

Thus, it has been possible to determine three mechanisms by which life increases chemical diversity: families of BGCs have the capacity to evolve from the merger of small subgroups that function as independent evolutionary entities (with families that have more than 1000 members); a large number of enzymes of the class polyketide synthases and nonribosomal peptide synthetases evolve together to facilitate chemical innovation; and BGCs can evolve using indistinctly different pathways individually, which causes greater versatility in the modulation of the response to the different environmental challenges (Cimermancic et al., 2014; Medema, Cimermancic, Sali, Takano, & Fischbach, 2014). The configuration of the BGCs as symbiogenome and hologenomes capable of establishing the interactions in the biocenosis confers on them a fundamental role in the adaptive evolution of the species and in the acquisition of complexity of the biological systems (Provorov, Tikhonovich, & Vorobyov, 2016). In this way, processes such as gene remodeling have been reported in prokaryotes, where it has been possible to observe the transfer of DNA fragments, as well as the acquisition of genetic material and its rearrangement, causing the evolution of composite genes with a greater number of adaptive functions (Méheust et al., 2018; Okada & Seyedsayamdost, 2017). One of the processes related to prokaryotes with this remodeling is the horizontal gene transfer that, through the mechanisms of conjugation, transformation, and transduction, has been used to form a network of innovation and information transfer for survival (Chu, Sprouffske, & Wagner, 2018; Soucy, Huang, & Gogarten, 2015). Finally, this gene transfer will result in a phenotypic transformation within the holobiont, constituting a fundamental co-evolution unit of the different metaorganisms and their ecosystems (Sitaraman, 2018). For this reason, the analysis of the evolution of the symbiotic holobiont will be a subject of study that will lead us to a redefinition of life as cooperative complexity and not as individuality (Sandoval-Motta, Aldana, & Frank, 2017).

1.7 Complex biological systems, cooperation, and solidarity

The use of systemism is perhaps the most useful and versatile way of understanding the diversity present in the biosphere, as well as the interactions that increase its chemical diversity (Bunge, 2017). These systems can also explain the functionality of cooperation phenomena such as symbiosis and episymbiosis (symbionts associated with the surface of the host) (Castelle & Banfield, 2018). It also delves into the description of the thermodynamic flow of the energy of the systems under the different sources used by life on earth in their evolutionary stages, such as geochemical energy, sunlight, oxygen, flesh, and fire (Judson, 2017). This is evidence of the strong correlation that exists between physical processes with the origin and maintenance of life (Tecon & Or, 2017). Thus, we see that biological systems, being products of evolution, diversify into the novelty of adaptation and make the system acquire the character of a biological unit in itself (Moreno & Mossio, 2015). In this way, the biological units described evolve as their ecological interactions evolve, modifying the inheritance of the biological systems in the construction of the niches; this notion of evolutionary ecology (evo-eco) contemplates the change as a result of the search of the dynamic homeostasis of the ecosystems. Although this concept talks about connection, it is more appropriate to talk about integration (Watson et al., 2016).

Under this molecular evolution for adaptation—partly Lamarckian for the machinery that involves host populations and partly Darwinian for its ability to select systems that recognize and learn—the systems acquire complexity and specialization, but they do not lose cooperation; that is, the rupture of homeostasis is the loss of cooperation and solidarity within the biological systems (Müller, de Boer, Bonhoeffer, & Szathmáry, 2018). This is a fundamental aspect, because each system persists to the extent that it possesses a greater degree of evolvability—defined as the capacity of the biological system to accumulate evolutionary changes of its living beings—because this makes them more prone to adaptation and this is only possible in the degree of the present interaction (Janković & Ćirković, 2016). But an important factor to take into consideration is the fundamental role that regulation must play within the system, because these mechanisms guarantee stability and sustainability; this is how these second-order mechanisms are not part of basic metabolic functions, but serve the purpose of maintaining an organization in chemical equilibrium (Bich, Mossio, Ruiz-Mirazo, & Moreno, 2016).

This is where we return to the notion of secondary metabolism as a primordial part of the biological system with the function of maintaining homeostasis and interaction within an ecosystem for adaptation and evolution (Hardoim et al., 2015). It is more to be observed that the establishment of a metabolic network within the ecological niche in co-evolution depends on and can only be optimized from the production of secondary metabolites that facilitate the reproductive and nutritional processes of the living beings that make up the biological system (Pande & Kost, 2017). For this reason, the secondary metabolism acquires great value as a symbiotic strategy that allows the development of symbiotic interactions within the holobiont and increases the evolvability of the biological system (Van der Meij, Worsley, Hutchings, & van Wezel, 2017). Finally, the transmission of information is what characterizes any successful biological system, by the acquisition of a greater evolutionary potential capable of granting the following generations of living beings the ability to continue cooperating in the biocenosis; all this by regulating the drivers of evolutionary innovation: reproduction, inheritance, variation, and interaction (Baquero, 2017). Likewise, nongenetic inheritance plays a crucial role in the evolution of populations in order to cope with rapidly changing environmental changes, and this process also facilitates genetic adaptation and the preservation of the system of genetic variation (O'Dea, Noble, Johnson, Hesselson, & Nakagawa, 2016).

On the other hand, it is necessary to take into consideration that the biological systems in cooperation and interaction must have the capacity to learn and to accumulate information on patterns of behavior in order to assume the phenotypic change in order to address the adaptive challenges of the ecosystem (Power et al., 2015). It is under this concept of evolutionary development (evo-devo) that phenotypic plasticity becomes the preparation of the genetic changes to the interior of the system necessary for the construction of the niche; as a consequence of this amalgam of processes. The interaction rises as one of the great evolutionary drivers (Müller, 2017).

1.8 Biotechnology of molecular evolution: Interaction in the application

The symbiotic interactions between organisms are what define their evolution and development, so the paradigm of unique species as productive units in biotechnology must be transformed into a model of integration of the communities (Ramanan, Kim, Cho, Oh, & Kim, 2016). In this way, the possibility of implementing models of metabolic communities based on their evolutionary interactions is a novel approach that can be applied to environmental and industrial biotechnology (Perez-Garcia, Lear, & Singhal, 2016). Likewise, the determination of the metabolic phenotypes that regulate the interactions of an organism with its environment and other living beings will be subject to study for application for industrial biochemistry and new drugs discovery (Machado, Andrejev, Tramontano, & Patil, 2018), as the present book poses. This approach to the search for an interactome as a biological system may be useful in understanding the homeostasis of the secondary metabolism in the holobiont and its role in disease, evolution, and transfer of information (Cortese-Krott et al., 2017). Similarly, the holobionts as a multicellular organization of the four domains (Prokaryota, Archaea, Eukaryota, and the Virome) are constituted as the phenomenon of macroorganic life that can interact with these models of communities seeking to constitute a biotechnology of the whole (Miller Jr. & Torday, 2018). In addition, the analysis of the different layers of the holobionic entity, such as the hologenome, the epigenome, and the metagenome, must be included as functional agents in the homeostasis of the system; but it is also important not to rule out the cognitive capacity of these complexities, because it will determine its evolutionary capacity for each applied model (Miller, 2016).

1.9 Conclusions

The configuration of a interactome in molecular evolution allows the speciation of living beings for the acquisition of degrees of complexity of an ecological niche; in this way, the metabolic networks that are established are the basis of adaptation by increasing the evolvability in character by the interactions that guarantee reproduction and nutrition. This is how, in this symbiogenesis, the secondary metabolism appears as an evolutionary tool for the regulation of the functions exerted by the primary metabolism, which acquires chemical diversity as it increases its biological activity. For this reason, the greater the degree of complexity, the higher the amount of metabolic interactions present. In this way, the implementation of novel biotechnological models based on the metabolic networks developed by the evolution of organisms within the biosphere is a manner of reaching new approaches that allow us to obtain and study useful holobionic entities in industrial biochemistry and biomedicine.

Acknowledgments

The author wants to thank P.S. Bird for his accompaniment and wise advice in ecosystem niches during the writing of this chapter.

References

Allard, P. M., Bisson, J., Azzollini, A., Pauli, G. F., Cordell, G. A., & Wolfender, J. L. (2018). Pharmacognosy in the digital era: Shifting to contextualized metabolomics. *Current Opinion in Biotechnology*, *54*, 57–64.

Andras, P., & Andras, C. (2005). The origins of life–the 'protein interaction world' hypothesis: Protein interactions were the first form of self-reproducing life and nucleic acids evolved later as memory molecules. *Medical Hypotheses*, *64*(4), 678–688.

Arnold, F. H. (2015). The nature of chemical innovation: New enzymes by evolution. *Quarterly Reviews of Biophysics*, *48*(4), 404–410.

Bang, C., Dagan, T., Deines, P., Dubilier, N., Duschl, W. J., Fraune, S., … Picazo, D. (2018). Metaorganisms in extreme environments: Do microbes play a role in organismal adaptation? *Zoology*, *127*(1), 1–19.

Bapteste, E., & Huneman, P. (2018). Toward a dynamic interaction network of life to unify and expand the evolutionary theory. *BMC Biology*, *16*(1), 56.

Baquero, F. (2017). Transmission as a basic process in microbial biology. Lwoff award prize lecture. *FEMS Microbiology Reviews*, *41*(6), 816–827.

Barge, L. M., Branscomb, E., Brucato, J. R., Cardoso, S. S. S., Cartwright, J. H. E., Danielache, S. O., … Robinson, K. J. (2017). Thermodynamics, disequilibrium, evolution: Far-from-equilibrium geological and chemical considerations for origin-of-life research. *Origins of Life and Evolution of Biospheres*, *47*(1), 39–56.

Bich, L., Mossio, M., Ruiz-Mirazo, K., & Moreno, A. (2016). Biological regulation: Controlling the system from within. *Biology and Philosophy*, *31*(2), 237–265.

Bordenstein, S. R., & Theis, K. R. (2015). Host biology in light of the microbiome: Ten principles of holobionts and hologenomes. *PLoS Biology*, *13*(8), e1002226.

Bosch, T. C., & McFall-Ngai, M. J. (2011). Metaorganisms as the new frontier. *Zoology*, *114*(4), 185–190.

Brockman, K. L., Azzari, P. N., Branstool, M. T., Atack, J. M., Schulz, B. L., Jen, F. E. C., … Bakaletz, L. O. (2018). Epigenetic regulation alters biofilm architecture and composition in multiple clinical isolates of nontypeable Haemophilus influenzae. *mBio*, *9*(5), e01682-18.

Bunge, M. (2017). Systemism: The alternative to individualism and holism. In H. Meadwell (Ed.), *The social sciences and rationality* (pp. 121–136). Routledge.

Carmona, D., Fitzpatrick, C. R., & Johnson, M. T. (2015). Fifty years of co-evolution and beyond: Integrating co-evolution from molecules to species. *Molecular Ecology*, *24*(21), 5315–5329.

Casadesús, J., & Low, D. A. (2013). Programmed heterogeneity: Epigenetic mechanisms in bacteria. *Journal of Biological Chemistry*, *288*(20), 13929–13935.

Castelle, C. J., & Banfield, J. F. (2018). Major new microbial groups expand diversity and alter our understanding of the tree of life. *Cell*, *172*(6), 1181–1197.

Chandel, N. S. (2015). Evolution of mitochondria as signaling organelles. *Cell Metabolism*, *22*(2), 204–206.

Chevin, L. M., & Beckerman, A. P. (2012). From adaptation to molecular evolution. *Heredity*, *108*(4), 457.

Chiu, L., & Gilbert, S. F. (2015). The birth of the holobiont: Multi-species birthing through mutual scaffolding and niche construction. *Biosemiotics*, *8*(2), 191–210.

Chu, H. Y., Sprouffske, K., & Wagner, A. (2018). Assessing the benefits of horizontal gene transfer by laboratory evolution and genome sequencing. *BMC Evolutionary Biology*, *18*(1), 54.

Cimermancic, P., Medema, M. H., Claesen, J., Kurita, K., Brown, L. C. W., Mavrommatis, K., … Birren, B. W. (2014). Insights into secondary metabolism from a global analysis of prokaryotic biosynthetic gene clusters. *Cell*, *158*(2), 412–421.

Clarke, E. (2016). Levels of selection in biofilms: Multispecies biofilms are not evolutionary individuals. *Biology and Philosophy*, *31*(2), 191–212.

Cleaves, H. J. (2018). Nucleobases on the primitive earth: Their sources and stabilities. In C. Menor-Salván (Ed.), *Prebiotic chemistry and chemical evolution of nucleic acids* (pp. 1–19). Cham: Springer.

Cortese-Krott, M. M., Koning, A., Kuhnle, G. G., Nagy, P., Bianco, C. L., Pasch, A., … Olson, K. R. (2017). The reactive species interactome: Evolutionary emergence, biological significance, and opportunities for redox metabolomics and personalized medicine. *Antioxidants & Redox Signaling*, *27*(10), 684–712.

De Loof, A. (2017). The evolution of "life": A Metadarwinian integrative approach. *Communicative & Integrative Biology*, *10*(3), e1301335.

De Tiège, A. (2017). The origins and physical roots of life's dual–metabolic and genetic–nature. *Life Science Press*, *1*(1), 31–39.

Detrain, C., & Deneubourg, J. L. (2006). Self-organized structures in a superorganism: Do ants "behave" like molecules? *Physics of Life Reviews*, *3*(3), 162–187.

Doolittle, W. F., & Booth, A. (2017). It's the song, not the singer: An exploration of holobiosis and evolutionary theory. *Biology and Philosophy*, *32*(1), 5–24.

Douglas, A. E. (2018). *Fundamentals of microbiome science: How microbes shape animal biology*. Princeton University Press.

Egbert, M. D., Barandiaran, X. E., & Di Paolo, E. A. (2011). Behavioral metabolution: The adaptive and evolutionary potential of metabolism-based chemotaxis. *Artificial Life*, *18*(1), 1–25.

Ekstig, B. (2015). Complexity, natural selection and the evolution of life and humans. *Foundations of Science*, *20*(2), 175–187.

Eskov, V. M., Filatova, O. E., Eskov, V. V., & Gavrilenko, T. V. (2017). The evolution of the idea of homeostasis: Determinism, stochastics, and chaos–self-organization. *Biophysics*, *62*(5), 809–820.

Even-Tov, E., Bendori, S. O., Valastyan, J., Ke, X., Pollak, S., Bareia, T., … Eldar, A. (2016). Social evolution selects for redundancy in bacterial quorum sensing. *PLoS Biology*, *14*(2), e1002386.

Fenzl, N. (2018). Emergence and self-organization of complex systems: The role of energy flows and information a philosophical approach. *Complexitas—Revista de Filosofia Temática*, *2*(1), 31–45.

Firn, R. D., & Jones, C. G. (2000). The evolution of secondary metabolism–a unifying model. *Molecular Microbiology*, *37*(5), 989–994.

Flemming, H. C., Wingender, J., Szewzyk, U., Steinberg, P., Rice, S. A., & Kjelleberg, S. (2016). Biofilms: An emergent form of bacterial life. *Nature Reviews Microbiology*, *14*(9), 563.

Fröhlich-Nowoisky, J., Kampf, C. J., Weber, B., Huffman, J. A., Pöhlker, C., Andreae, M. O., … Su, H. (2016). Bioaerosols in the earth system: Climate, health, and ecosystem interactions. *Atmospheric Research*, *182*, 346–376.

Futuyma, D. J., & Agrawal, A. A. (2009). Macroevolution and the biological diversity of plants and herbivores. *Proceedings of the National Academy of Sciences*, https://doi.org/10.1073/pnas.0904106106.

Gilbert, S. F., Sapp, J., & Tauber, A. I. (2012). A symbiotic view of life: We have never been individuals. *The Quarterly Review of Biology*, *87*(4), 325–341.

Giordano, D., Coppola, D., Russo, R., Denaro, R., Giuliano, L., Lauro, F. M., ... Verde, C. (2015). Marine microbial secondary metabolites: Pathways, evolution and physiological roles. In R. K. Poole (Ed.), Vol. 66. *Advances in microbial physiology* (pp. 357–428). Academic Press.

Grzybowski, B. A., & Huck, W. T. (2016). The nanotechnology of life-inspired systems. *Nature Nanotechnology*, *11*(7), 585.

Guerrero, R., Margulis, L., & Berlanga, M. (2013). Symbiogenesis: The holobiont as a unit of evolution. *International Microbiology*, *16*(3), 133–143.

Haag, K. L. (2018). Holobionts and their hologenomes: Evolution with mixed modes of inheritance. *Genetics and Molecular Biology*, *41*(1 Suppl. 1), 189.

Hansen, S. K., Rainey, P. B., Haagensen, J. A., & Molin, S. (2007). Evolution of species interactions in a biofilm community. *Nature*, *445*(7127), 533.

Hardoim, P. R., Van Overbeek, L. S., Berg, G., Pirttilä, A. M., Compant, S., Campisano, A., ... Sessitsch, A. (2015). The hidden world within plants: Ecological and evolutionary considerations for defining functioning of microbial endophytes. *Microbiology and Molecular Biology Reviews*, *79*(3), 293–320.

Harms, M. J., & Thornton, J. W. (2013). Evolutionary biochemistry: Revealing the historical and physical causes of protein properties. *Nature Reviews Genetics*, *14*(8), 559.

Hochberg, M. E., Marquet, P. A., Boyd, R., & Wagner, A. (2017). Innovation: An emerging focus from cells to societies. *Philosophical Transactions of the Royal Society of London Series B, Biological Sciences*, *372*(1735).

Holovatch, Y., Kenna, R., & Thurner, S. (2017). Complex systems: Physics beyond physics. *European Journal of Physics*, *38*(2), 023002.

Hoogendoorn, K., Barra, L., Waalwijk, C., Dickschat, J. S., van der Lee, T. A., & Medema, M. H. (2018). Evolution and diversity of biosynthetic gene clusters in Fusarium. *Frontiers in Microbiology*, *9*.

Hordijk, W., Naylor, J., Krasnogor, N., & Fellermann, H. (2018). Population dynamics of autocatalytic sets in a compartmentalized spatial world. *Life*, *8*(3), 33.

Jacobs, W. M., & Frenkel, D. (2016). Self-assembly of structures with addressable complexity. *Journal of the American Chemical Society*, *138*(8), 2457–2467.

Janković, S., & Ćirković, M. M. (2016). Evolvability is an evolved ability: The coding concept as the arch-unit of natural selection. *Origins of Life and Evolution of Biospheres*, *46*(1), 67–79.

Jenke-Kodama, H., Müller, R., & Dittmann, E. (2008). Evolutionary mechanisms underlying secondary metabolite diversity. In F. Petersen & R. Amstutz (Eds.), Vol. I. *Natural compounds as drugs* (pp. 119–140). Basel: Birkhäuser.

Jorgenson, T. D., Mohammed, A. M., Agrawal, D. K., & Schulman, R. (2017). Self-assembly of hierarchical DNA nanotube architectures with well-defined geometries. *ACS Nano*, *11*(2), 1927–1936.

Judson, O. P. (2017). The energy expansions of evolution. *Nature Ecology & Evolution*, *1*(6), 0138.

Katsnelson, M. I., Wolf, Y. I., & Koonin, E. V. (2018). Towards physical principles of biological evolution. *Physica Scripta*, *93*(4), 043001.

Kleidon, A., Malhi, Y., & Cox, P. M. (2010). Maximum entropy production in environmental and ecological systems. *Philosophical Transactions of the Royal Society, B: Biological Sciences*, *365*(1545), 1297.

Kragh, K. N., Hutchison, J. B., Melaugh, G., Rodesney, C., Roberts, A. E., Irie, Y., ... Bjarnsholt, T. (2016). Role of multicellular aggregates in biofilm formation. *MBio*, 7(2), e00237-16.

Krishnamurthy, R. (2017). Giving rise to life: Transition from prebiotic chemistry to protobiology. *Accounts of Chemical Research*, *50*(3), 455–459.

Lerat, E., & Moran, N. A. (2004). The evolutionary history of quorum-sensing systems in bacteria. *Molecular Biology and Evolution*, *21*(5), 903–913.

Longo, G., Montévil, M., & Kauffman, S. (2012, July). *No entailing laws, but enablement in the evolution of the biosphere*. In: *Proceedings of the 14th annual conference companion on genetic and evolutionary computation*.ACM. (pp. 1379–1392).

Longo, G., Montévil, M., Sonnenschein, C., & Soto, A. M. (2015). In search of principles for a theory of organisms. *Journal of Biosciences*, *40*(5), 955–968.

López-Maury, L., Marguerat, S., & Bähler, J. (2008). Tuning gene expression to changing environments: From rapid responses to evolutionary adaptation. *Nature Reviews Genetics*, *9*(8), 583.

Love, A. C. (2015). Evolutionary developmental biology: Philosophical issues. In T. H. Philippe, H. Guillaume, & L. M. Silberstein (Eds.), *Handbook of evolutionary thinking in the sciences* (pp. 265–283). Dordrecht: Springer.

Lyons, N. A., & Kolter, R. (2015). On the evolution of bacterial multicellularity. *Current Opinion in Microbiology*, *24*, 21–28.

Ma'ayan, A. (2017). Complex systems biology. *Journal of the Royal Society Interface*, *14*(134), 20170391.

Machado, D., Andrejev, S., Tramontano, M., & Patil, K. R. (2018). Fast automated reconstruction of genome-scale metabolic models for microbial species and communities. *Nucleic Acids Research*, *46*(15), 7542–7553.

Maciá, E. (2005). The role of aperiodic order in science and technology. *Reports on Progress in Physics*, *69*(2), 397.

Massey, S. E., & Mishra, B. (2018). Origin of biomolecular games: Deception and molecular evolution. *Journal of the Royal Society Interface*, *15*(146), 20180429.

Mayer, C., Schreiber, U., & Dávila, M. J. (2015). Periodic vesicle formation in tectonic fault zones—An ideal scenario for molecular evolution. *Origins of Life and Evolution of Biospheres*, *45*(1–2), 139–148.

Mayer, C., Schreiber, U., & Dávila, M. J. (2017). Selection of prebiotic molecules in amphiphilic environments. *Life*, 7(1), 3.

Medema, M. H., Cimermancic, P., Sali, A., Takano, E., & Fischbach, M. A. (2014). A systematic computational analysis of biosynthetic gene cluster evolution: Lessons for engineering biosynthesis. *PLoS Computational Biology*, *10*(12), e1004016.

Méheust, R., Watson, A. K., Lapointe, F. J., Papke, R. T., Lopez, P., & Bapteste, E. (2018). Hundreds of novel composite genes and chimeric genes with bacterial origins contributed to haloarchaeal evolution. *Genome Biology*, *19*(1), 75.

Melkikh, A. V. (2014). Quantum information and the problem of mechanisms of biological evolution. *Biosystems*, *115*, 33–45.

Miller, W. B. (2016). Cognition, information fields and hologenomic entanglement: Evolution in light and shadow. *Biology*, *5*(2), 21.

Miller, W. B., Jr., & Torday, J. S. (2018). Four domains: The fundamental unicell and post-Darwinian cognition-based evolution. *Progress in Biophysics and Molecular Biology*, *140*, 49–73.

Moreno, A., & Mossio, M. (2015). *Evolution: The historical dimension of autonomy*. In *Biological autonomy*. Dordrecht: Springer. (pp. 111–139).

Moreno-Gámez, S., Sorg, R. A., Domenech, A., Kjos, M., Weissing, F. J., Doorn, G. S., & Veening, J. W. (2017). Quorum sensing integrates environmental cues, cell density and cell history to control bacterial competence. *Nature Communications*, *8*(1), 854.

Müller, G. B. (2017). Why an extended evolutionary synthesis is necessary. *Interface focus*, 7(5), 20170015.

Müller, V., de Boer, R. J., Bonhoeffer, S., & Szathmáry, E. (2018). An evolutionary perspective on the systems of adaptive immunity. *Biological Reviews*, *93*(1), 505–528.

Muraille, E. (2018). Diversity generator mechanisms are essential components of biological systems: The two queen hypothesis. *Frontiers in Microbiology*, *9*, 223.

Murr, L. E. (2015). Aperiodic crystal structures: Quasicrystals. In L. E. Murr (Ed.), *Handbook of materials structures, properties, processing and performance* (pp. 183–192). Cham: Springer.

Nguyen, L., Lang, D., van Gessel, N., Beike, A. K., Menges, A., Reski, R., & Roth-Nebelsick, A. (2016). Evolutionary processes as models for exploratory design. In J. Knippers, K. G. Nickel, & T. Speck (Eds.), *Biomimetic research for architecture and building construction* (pp. 295–318). Cham: Springer.

O'Malley, M. A. (2017). From endosymbiosis to holobionts: Evaluating a conceptual legacy. *Journal of Theoretical Biology*, *434*, 34–41.

O'Dea, R. E., Noble, D. W. A., Johnson, S. L., Hesselson, D., & Nakagawa, S. (2016). The role of non-genetic inheritance in evolutionary rescue: Epigenetic buffering, heritable bet hedging and epigenetic traps. *Environmental Epigenetics*, *2*(1), dvv014.

Okada, B. K., & Seyedsayamdost, M. R. (2017). Antibiotic dialogues: Induction of silent biosynthetic gene clusters by exogenous small molecules. *FEMS Microbiology Reviews*, *41*(1), 19–33.

Pande, S., & Kost, C. (2017). Bacterial unculturability and the formation of intercellular metabolic networks. *Trends in Microbiology*, *25*(5), 349–361.

Perez-Garcia, O., Lear, G., & Singhal, N. (2016). Metabolic network modeling of microbial interactions in natural and engineered environmental systems. *Frontiers in Microbiology*, 7, 673.

Picard, M., & Burelle, Y. (2012). Mitochondria: Starving to reach quorum? Insight into the physiological purpose of mitochondrial fusion. *BioEssays*, *34*(4), 272–274.

Polesskaya, O., Guschin, V., Kondratev, N., Garanina, I., Nazarenko, O., Zyryanova, N., … Zhao, Y. (2018). On possible role of DNA electrodynamics in chromatin regulation. *Progress in Biophysics and Molecular Biology*, *30*, 1e5.

Power, D. A., Watson, R. A., Szathmáry, E., Mills, R., Powers, S. T., Doncaster, C. P., & Czapp, B. (2015). What can ecosystems learn? Expanding evolutionary ecology with learning theory. *Biology Direct*, *10*(1), 69.

Provorov, N. A., Tikhonovich, I. A., & Vorobyov, N. I. (2016). Symbiogenesis as a model for reconstructing the early stages of genome evolution. *Russian Journal of Genetics*, *52*(2), 117–124.

Ramanan, R., Kim, B. H., Cho, D. H., Oh, H. M., & Kim, H. S. (2016). Algae–bacteria interactions: Evolution, ecology and emerging applications. *Biotechnology Advances*, *34*(1), 14–29.

Ren, Y., & You, L. (2015). Dynamic signaling cascades: Reversible covalent reaction-coupled molecular switches. *Journal of the American Chemical Society*, *137*(44), 14220–14228.

Rosenberg, E., & Zilber-Rosenberg, I. (2018). The hologenome concept of evolution after 10 years. *Microbiome*, *6*(1), 78.

Sandoval-Motta, S., Aldana, M., & Frank, A. (2017). Evolving ecosystems: Inheritance and selection in the light of the microbiome. *Archives of Medical Research*, *48*(8), 780–789.

Sardanyés, J., Lázaro, J. T., Guillamon, A., & Fontich, E. (2017). Full analysis of small hypercycles with short-circuits in prebiotic evolution. *Physica D: Nonlinear Phenomena*, *347*, 90–108.

Schluter, J., Schoech, A. P., Foster, K. R., & Mitri, S. (2016). The evolution of quorum sensing as a mechanism to infer kinship. *PLoS Computational Biology*, *12*(4), e1004848.

Sevim, S., Sorrenti, A., Franco, C., Furukawa, S., Pané, S., & Puigmartí-Luis, J. (2018). Self-assembled materials and supramolecular chemistry within microfluidic environments: From common thermodynamic states to non-equilibrium structures. *Chemical Society Reviews*, *47*(11), 3788–3803.

Sharov, A. A. (2014). Evolutionary constraints or opportunities? *Biosystems*, *123*, 9–18.

Shepelin, D., Hansen, A., Lennen, R., Luo, H., & Herrgård, M. (2018). Selecting the best: Evolutionary engineering of chemical production in microbes. *Genes*, *9*(5), 249.

Sitaraman, R. (2018). Prokaryotic horizontal gene transfer within the human holobiont: Ecological-evolutionary inferences, implications and possibilities. *Microbiome*, *6*(1), 163.

Soucy, S. M., Huang, J., & Gogarten, J. P. (2015). Horizontal gene transfer: Building the web of life. *Nature Reviews Genetics*, *16*(8), 472.

Spitzer, J., Pielak, G. J., & Poolman, B. (2015). Emergence of life: Physical chemistry changes the paradigm. *Biology Direct*, *10*(1), 33.

Spitzer, J., & Poolman, B. (2009). The role of biomacromolecular crowding, ionic strength, and physicochemical gradients in the complexities of life's emergence. *Microbiology and Molecular Biology Reviews*, *73*(2), 371–388.

Steenackers, H. P., Parijs, I., Foster, K. R., & Vanderleyden, J. (2016). Experimental evolution in biofilm populations. *FEMS Microbiology Reviews*, *40*(3), 373–397.

Strogatz, S. H. (2018). *Nonlinear dynamics and chaos: With applications to physics, biology, chemistry, and engineering*. CRC Press.

Sun, L., & Wu, R. (2015). Mapping complex traits as a dynamic system. *Physics of Life Reviews*, *13*, 155–185.

Tecon, R., & Or, D. (2017). Biophysical processes supporting the diversity of microbial life in soil. *FEMS Microbiology Reviews*, *41*(5), 599–623.

Tëmkin, I., & Eldredge, N. (2015). Networks and hierarchies: Approaching complexity in evolutionary theory. In E. Serrelli & N. Gontier (Eds.), *Macroevolution* (pp. 183–226). Cham: Springer.

Tianero, M. D., Pierce, E., Raghuraman, S., Sardar, D., McIntosh, J. A., Heemstra, J. R., … Bachmann, B. O. (2016). Metabolic model for diversity-generating biosynthesis. *Proceedings of the National Academy of Sciences*, *113*(7), 1772–1777.

Tkačik, G., & Bialek, W. (2016). Information processing in living systems. *Annual Review of Condensed Matter Physics*, 7, 89–117.

Torday, J. S., & Miller, W. B. (2016). Phenotype as agent for epigenetic inheritance. *Biology*, *5*(3), 30.

Van Der Heijden, M. G., Bardgett, R. D., & Van Straalen, N. M. (2008). The unseen majority: Soil microbes as drivers of plant diversity and productivity in terrestrial ecosystems. *Ecology Letters*, *11*(3), 296–310.

Van der Meij, A., Worsley, S. F., Hutchings, M. I., & van Wezel, G. P. (2017). Chemical ecology of antibiotic production by actinomycetes. *FEMS Microbiology Reviews*, *41*(3), 392–416.

Varn, D. P., & Crutchfield, J. P. (2016). What did Erwin mean? The physics of information from the materials genomics of aperiodic crystals and water to molecular information catalysts and life. *Philosophical Transactions of the Royal Society A*, *374*(2063), 20150067.

Wagner, A., & Rosen, W. (2014). Spaces of the possible: Universal Darwinism and the wall between technological and biological innovation. *Journal of the Royal Society Interface*, *11*(97), 20131190.

Walker, S. I. (2017). Origins of life: A problem for physics, a key issues review. *Reports on Progress in Physics*, *80*(9), 092601.

Watson, R. A., Mills, R., Buckley, C. L., Kouvaris, K., Jackson, A., Powers, S. T., … Power, D. (2016). Evolutionary connectionism: Algorithmic principles underlying the evolution of biological organisation in evo-devo, evo-eco and evolutionary transitions. *Evolutionary Biology*, *43*(4), 553–581.

Wills, P. R. (2016). DNA as information. *Philosophical Transactions of the Royal Society A*, *374*(2063), 20150417.

Wu, G., Yan, Q., Jones, J. A., Tang, Y. J., Fong, S. S., & Koffas, M. A. (2016). Metabolic burden: Cornerstones in synthetic biology and metabolic engineering applications. *Trends in Biotechnology*, *34*(8), 652–664.

Zenil, H. (2013). Turing patterns with Turing machines: Emergence and low-level structure formation. *Natural Computing*, *12*(2), 291–303.

Zilber-Rosenberg, I., & Rosenberg, E. (2008). Role of microorganisms in the evolution of animals and plants: The hologenome theory of evolution. *FEMS Microbiology Reviews*, *32*(5), 723–735.

Zwart, H. (2018). Scientific iconoclasm and active imagination: Synthetic cells as technoscientific mandalas. *Life Sciences, Society and Policy*, *14*(1), 10.

CHAPTER 2

Thermodynamics of secondary metabolism: The triumph of living systems

Man at last knows he is alone in the unfeeling immensity of the universe, out of which he has emerged only by chance. His destiny is nowhere spelled out, nor is his duty. The kingdom above or the darkness below; it is for him to choose

Jacques Monod (1910–76)

The origin of life has been one of the deepest deadlocks of Darwinism. A century of scientific research - and common sense - reveal that there are no mechanisms or laws in nature to organize simple molecules into a living cell. In fact as the Second Law of Thermodynamics proposes, the molecules on Earth would naturally tend to disorganize; which means an increase in entropy.

Ilya Prigogine (1917–2003)

2.1 Introduction

Because life, as a complex system, obeys the laws of thermodynamics, which regulate both primary and secondary metabolism in living beings in evolution (Mossio & Bich, 2017; Pereira, Vimal, & Pregnolato, 2017), this is how the secondary metabolism appears as a teleonomic mechanism that allows the functions of the primary metabolism in cells in the replicative state (Pross, 2004, 2005). It is in this order of ideas that life acquires its autocatalytic character, through the establishment of a metabolism of bioactive molecules that allow cells to acquire nutrients and survive environmental changes (Baverstock, 2013). Such is the case with low-molecular-weight metabolites (LMWMs) that contribute to cellular respiration due to their role as electron donors, and with other varied functions such as nutrients, vitamins, hormones, scents, and antioxidants, as well as promising applications such as medicines and biopolymers (Hadacek & Bachmann, 2015).

Molecular Evolutionary Models in Drug Discovery
https://doi.org/10.1016/B978-0-12-817613-9.00002-X

In this way we can appreciate how the secondary metabolites help maintain the energy and material flows that the biological system requires (Metallo & Vander Heiden, 2013), maintaining the cell as an entity capable of self-renewing (Tessera, 2018). In addition, this autocatalytic functionality derived from compounds with adaptive biological activity is a critical evolutionary factor of the species (Harms & Thornton, 2013). Furthermore, this complex intermolecular network acquires a supramolecular state to achieve a homeostasis that allows for survival (Epstein, 2018), which leads the living organism to develop signaling and intercellular communication systems with which to establish an ecosystemic niche of cooperation (Raes & Bork, 2008; Trosko, 2016). Additionally, these communication channels cause the thermodynamic equilibrium of the biological system to be maintained by the exchange of information for adaptation (Tu & Rappel, 2018). It is also important to take into account the regulation of epigenetics on secondary metabolism and its implications of energy flow. This metaboloepigenetics is maintained in equilibrium by metabolites (Donohoe & Bultman, 2012); also, these cofactors have the ability to regulate epigenetic signals in the search for homeostasis (Meier, 2013; Metallo & Vander Heiden, 2010). This is how the bioenergetic processes that make up the holobionts finally establish the interactions between the different ecosystems (Bapteste & Huneman, 2018; zu Castell, Lüttge, & Matyssek, 2019).

Because of the above, the objective of this chapter is to provide a comprehensive vision that combines the evolution of biological systems with the thermodynamics of secondary metabolism in order to develop innovations that use the biophysical applications of thermodynamics to apply bioinspired models in the design of drugs with novel forms of distribution (Demetzos, 2015).

2.2 Life in the second law of thermodynamics

More than saying that life is a manifestation of the second law of thermodynamics, it is considered that life is a demonstration of the predictive capacity of the model described in the second law of thermodynamics (Bai, Ge, & Qian, 2018; Schlitter, 2018), because the fact of predicting that each biological phenomenon for the acquisition of energy is irreversible gives life a nuance of constant change that must remain and be sustained over time to achieve an evolutionary success (Miller Jr., 2018). Likewise, it predisposes to negentropy as a model, which explains the thermodynamic presence of secondary metabolism and its regulation as part of the fitness of organisms against environmental factors, as has been discovered in the natural production of antibiotics (Yan et al., 2018). So this coevolution within an interactome is what stimulates the chemical diversity within the metabolites (Speed, Fenton, Jones, Ruxton, & Brockhurst, 2015), being through these pluricellular interactomes of signaling and communication where entropy is exported throughout the ecosystem (Reen, McGlacken, & O'Gara, 2018; Tsuruyama, 2018). In addition, this regulatory role of biomolecules causes the speed of irreversible processes to change (Li & Snyder, 2011; Liu, Ma, Yuan, & Feng, 2018), given the asymmetry that biomolecules include within biochemical cycles to enrich diversity from the three basic components of life: organic molecules, liquid water, and energy (Aerts, Röling, Elsaesser, & Ehrenfreund, 2014). Thus, the application of regulatory metabolites leads to an increase in negentropy within a living organism, altering the speed of the energy process (Skene, 2015). This allows metabolic flexibility as a means to maintain energy homeostasis within the biological system (Smith, Soeters, Wüst, & Houtkooper, 2018). Likewise, this fluctuation between the environmental challenges and the adaptive responses that induce evolution are those that allow the system to go from phenotypic to genotypic changes (Fig. 1) (Kaneko & Furusawa, 2018), which could explain the diversity observed by the accumulation of adaptations in the biosynthetic gene clusters (BGCs), thanks to their eagerness to regulate toward a favorable balance of the energy flows (Du, Zielinski, Monk, & Palsson, 2018).

This search for thermodynamic equilibrium is what has established the presence of a hidden chemistry within BGCs, whose potential is only expressed by virtue of the survival needs of an ecosystem (Asplund-Samuelsson, Janasch, & Hudson, 2018; Cruz-Morales et al., 2016); of which it can be

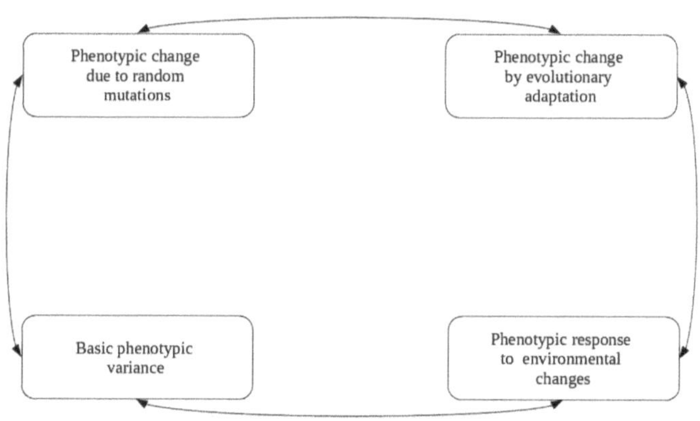

Fig. 1 Fluctuation between environmental changes and evolutionary adaptation.

deduced that not only the manipulation of the BGCs is necessary, it is also required that the system acquires a homeostasis so that this is expressed (Okada & Seyedsayamdost, 2017; Rigali, Anderssen, Naômé, & van Wezel, 2018). Therefore, it can be conjectured that the BGCs contain enough information to predict the environment in order to maintain the sustainability of complex biological systems (Seoane & Solé, 2018).

2.3 Thermodynamics of intercellular communication

In intercellular communication, information as well as negentropy is transferred by Brownian motion (Davies, Rieper, & Tuszynski, 2013; Eckford, Kuznets-Speck, Hinczewski, & Thomas, 2018). In this model of molecular communication, a molecule transmitter is required, a means of propagation within the ecosystem, the receiver and an encoded information, in order to share information for adaptation are required (Fig. 2) (Kadloor, Adve, & Eckford, 2012). This exchange in a complex biological system establishes a set of chemical reactions between ligand and receptor that is framed in the energy flow of the system (Femminella, Reali, & Vasilakos, 2015; Lancet, Zidovetzki, & Markovitch, 2018).

This is how, in this order of ideas, the protein metabolite interaction becomes possible to maintain a homeostatic regulation within the interactome of the biological cycles (Piazza et al., 2018). In this area, the sociomicrobiology regulated by the quorum sensing arises at the origin of life on earth (Keller & Surette, 2006; Lyon, 2007). This is how, in the evolution of

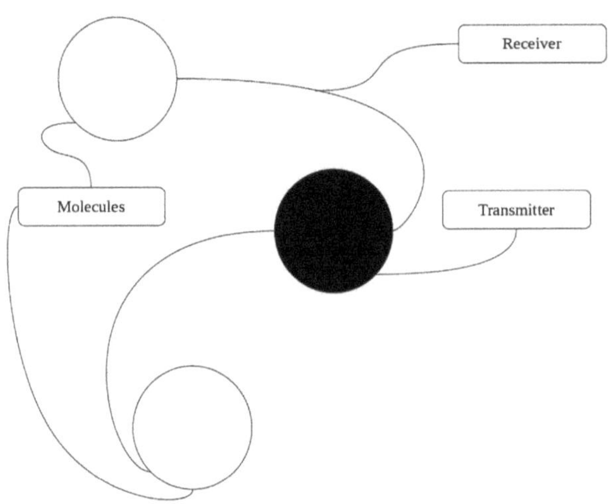

Fig. 2 Model of the molecular communication system.

molecular replicators, it was possible to establish a network of connection and transmission of information that persists with cell biology (Duim & Otto, 2017; Nee, 2016). Then the thermodynamic stability acquired by the first molecular replicators is still used to transfer entropy in biological systems (Piñero & Solé, 2018; Vitas & Dobovišek, 2018).

On the other hand, by assuming the living cell as a bioinformational entity, it has the capacity to use the molecular communication of the secondary metabolism to activate the responses of the communities, as well as its adaptive learning (Moral, González, Navarro, & Marijuán, 2011), this circulation of bioinformation in conjunction with entropy and free energy will end up defining the natural system and its evolution (Kompanichenko, 2014), all thanks to a dynamic of proteins based on irreversible thermodynamic changes that alter their conformation and functionality (Zhao, 2013). Equally, the metabolic fitness that cells acquire to survive as they mutate requires thermodynamic regulation to carry out an evolutionary process of success (Bajić, Vila, Blount, & Sánchez, 2018; Pinu et al., 2018), defining evolutionary success as the ability to transfer information to the next generation while maintaining the trend toward the production of maximum entropy (Koch & Britton, 2018).

2.4 Thermodynamic epigenetics of secondary metabolism

To obtain a principle of functionality in a biological system it is necessary to evaluate the different cellular components from the modification of the DNA, as well as its transcription and interaction with RNA, proteins, and metabolites (Basler, Fernie, & Nikoloski, 2018). This is how functionality is determined by the flow of metabolic acquisition of energy in the system (Dai & Locasale, 2018); in addition, the development and its epigenetic control is determined by metabolic state, an aspect known as the Warburg effect (Gándara & Wappner, 2018). So, in this carbon-based metabolism, there is a connection of regulation through cellular communications established as part of the sharing of entropy (Miyazawa & Aulehla, 2018; Naviaux, 2018). In this order of ideas, we can consider that the secondary metabolism influences the dissipation of energy in the catabolism of glucose (Zivieri & Pacini, 2018). Thus, the role of secondary metabolites, such as polyphenols and others produced by the microbiome (bile acids) in their action as bioactive compounds capable of regulating metabolism in thermogenesis, has been observed (Reynés, Palou, Rodríguez, & Palou, 2019), as well as increasing resilience against cell stress (Pasinetti et al., 2018).

Likewise, thermodynamics in the regulation of metabolic flux can explain the heterogeneity of cell development as well as the concentration of various metabolites (De Martino, Andersson, Bergmiller, Guet, & Tkačik, 2018; Fernandez-de-Cossio-Diaz & Mulet, 2019).

It is necessary to assume that there is a coevolution between the enzymes and the metabolites that allows the continued evolution of the metabolic networks. In this interaction, it is possible that the origination of new metabolites with a physiological function is through the recruitment after the appearance of new components due to environmental changes and the phenomenon of enzymatic promiscuity (Noda-Garcia, Liebermeister, & Tawfik, 2018). It is also important to take into account the role of riboswitches that respond to certain metabolites, which leads to a control of gene expression and transcription mediated by bioactive compounds (Sinumvayo, Zhao, & Tuyishime, 2018); this leads to the presence of a self-regulation of secondary metabolism in the biological networks mediated by feedback mechanisms (Baral, Akhgari, & Metsä-Ketelä, 2018). In addition, metabolite sensors help to maintain metabolic fluxes by regulating gene expression, which tries to bring the cell to thermodynamic stability (Planqué, Hulshof, Teusink, Hendriks, & Bruggeman, 2018). For this reason, the epigenetic regulation of the tendency to entropy allows the cell to maintain a balance in constant exchange with its biological system, and is a determining factor in the development of new alternatives for the treatment and prevention of disease (Corso-Díaz, Jaeger, Chaitankar, & Swaroop, 2018; Tarabichi et al., 2013). This regulation also favors the functional integrity of the system by sharing entropy through molecular communication by adaptation using secondary metabolism (Chen, 2018).

2.5 Symbiotic holobiont thermodynamics

Now the adaptive plasticity of an organism in the flow of energy will depend on its configuration as a holobiont and how it interacts in a symbiotic way with its biological system (Baedke, 2018; Gilbert, Bosch, & Ledón-Rettig, 2015), with the aim to carry out the transition toward a metasystem in which the thermodynamic flow acquires a connotation that makes the equilibrium possible in a coevolutionary phenomenon (Benavides-Mendoza, 2018; Last, 2015). This means that the consequent biological evolution of the holobiont is conditioned in a parallel way by the laws of thermodynamics (Hansen, Popovic, Tolley, & Woodfield, 2018), and consequently in the cycle conformed by energy, biological information and communication take cognition as self-reference (Miller Jr., 2018; Miller Jr. & Torday, 2018). Thus, in the holobiont, defined as a eukaryotic organism with an assembly of prokaryotes in symbiotic interaction, the negentropy is achieved to obtain an order within (Kutschera, 2018). Then, to reach the thermodynamic stability, the holobiont has to adaptively change the hologenome, considered as all the genetic content present in the living beings that make up the holobiont (Morris, 2018).

Taking into account that life is the state of self-consciousness that allows the modulation of conditions depending on the needs of the organism, it is important to state that the control of entropy induces the action of the holobionts belonging to a metasystem (Corning & Szathmáry, 2015; Miller, 2016). Establishing in the process a great chemical diversity that defines the whole of the interactome from and to the living organism (Kessler & Kalske, 2018), all this is in order to increase the capacity of anticipation and prediction of the multicellular organism to obtain resources and achieve a state of homeostasis that allows its survival (Miller Jr., Torday, & Baluška, 2018). Thus, the entropic interactome contributes to the molecular communication and the maintenance of the thermal flow in the biological system (Lambert et al., 2019; Li, Chavali, Pancsa, Chavali, & Babu, 2018). In addition, interactome versatility is permitted by the heterogeneity of proteins and their interactions fuzziness, which gives complexity to the system, but also will increase its ability to anticipate to environmental challenges (Maity et al., 2018; Petrakis & Andrade-Navarro, 2016). In this way, fuzziness of protein becomes a source of diversity and dynamics for the holobiont, which enables it to establish connections with the metasystem (Amedei & Boem, 2018; Muraille, 2018), and it is in this mutual support where this symbiotic association leads the holobiont and its hologenome to an evolution of its adaptive capacity to reach a thermodynamic equilibrium (Carrier & Reitzel, 2017; Simon, Marchesi, Mougel, & Selosse, 2019).

2.6 Entropic interactomes and their influence in the hologenome

Negentropy in symbiotic relationships establish stability among the elements of the holobiont (Voss, Leon, Dhurandhar, & Robb, 2015), being in this state as an ecological dynamic of communication and interaction with the other elements within the metasystem is acquired (Hurst, 2017). In this way, the biological systems increase the negentropy when establishing communications between their holobionts (Torday & Miller Jr., 2017), and in this coevolution of mutual support, phenotypic adaptation and epigenetic regulation end up leading to a transformation of the hologenome that increases fitness (Torday & Miller Jr., 2018). So the holobiont and its symbiotic interactions acquire their position as a unit of selection that proliferates in conjunction with their exo- and endosymbionts (Hutzil, Sandoval-Motta, Frank, & Aldana, 2018; Roughgarden, Gilbert, Rosenberg, Zilber-Rosenberg, & Lloyd, 2018). Then one might ask how the hologenome mutates as the molecular interactions of holobiont evolve. This could be due to three primary factors: modulation of populations within the holobiont microbiome, acquisition of new microorganism, and horizontal transfer of genes from the microbiome to the host's genome (Rosenberg & Zilber-Rosenberg, 2018, 2019).

Thus, the changes in an evolutionary context in the holobiont exerted by its microbiome are directly on the phenotype and indirectly on the genotype (Sitaraman, 2018). These associations depend on the chemical information with which the symbiotic microorganisms participate in the communication signals in the host, which has been called the fermentation hypothesis (Carthey, Gillings, & Blumstein, 2018). In this exchange of small communicating molecules both the thermodynamic equilibrium and dysbiosis are at stake, as well as homeostasis and disease (Cleary, Condren, Zink, & Sanchez, 2017). This establishes an integrative model of the diversity of chemical signaling as a fundamental factor of evolution (Fig. 3) (Brunetti et al., 2018), an evolution that is consolidated through the formation of molecular networks of information that interconnects the

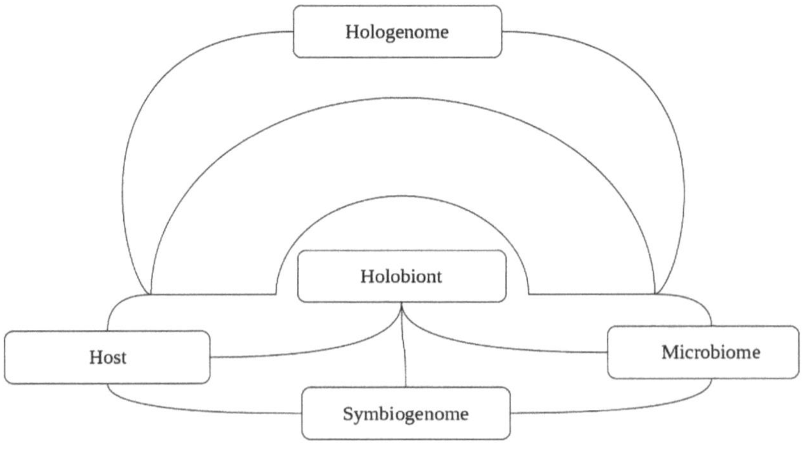

Fig. 3 Interactions inside holobiont.

metasystem in its entirety (Bapteste & Huneman, 2018). Entropy, communication, mutation, and evolution are the fundamental pillars of biological systems (Porcar, 2019).

2.7 Biosynthetic gene clusters: Communication and entropy

To establish a community of self-sustaining organisms in constant dynamics, it is necessary to have interaction and exchange paths of the energy flow of the system (Kong, Meldgin, Collins, & Lu, 2018). So, under this principle of free energy, organisms tend to self-organize by means of active inference (Kirchhoff, Parr, Palacios, Friston, & Kiverstein, 2018). In order to establish communication and interaction, the organisms contain a group of genes called biosynthetic gene clusters (BGCs) that express biochemically active metabolites, as well as the presence of combinatorial chemical biosynthesis processes within the BGCs through subclusters, which provides them with greater diversity and versatility (Del Carratore et al., 2019). In addition, these groups of genes are epigenetically regulated depending on the interactions of the organism with its environment (Colinas & Goossens, 2018; Keller, 2018). Likewise, BGCs help the holobionts in their symbiotic relationships and share entropy with the other members of the biological system (Rosenberg, Sharon, Atad, & Zilber-Rosenberg, 2010). This is how the biosynthetic gene clusters acquire diversity of information in the search for homeostasis and this happens as much in the human holobiont as in other ecosystems (Donia et al., 2014; Hoogendoorn et al., 2018).

In this way, BGCs, as important elements of the hologenome, also modulate the evolution of the host in its constant interaction with the biological system (Mendoza et al., 2018; Sharon et al., 2014). Likewise, this biological adaptation of the hologenome mediated by BGCs has achieved the constant evolution of eukaryotic organisms, due to its relationship with its microbial symbionts (Douglas, 2014; Moran & Sloan, 2015). Then the symbiosis of the hologenome within the interactome is a factor that increases the negentropy of the system and allows the survival of the organism that adapts (Catania et al., 2017). Finally, the holobiont acquires fitness due to the production, regulation, and recombination of the different secondary metabolites that are expressed in the BGCs and, in this exchange of chemical information, the hologenome mutates toward a new state of equilibrium (Patra, Schluttenhofer, Wu, Pattanaik, & Yuan, 2013).

2.8 Thermodynamics in complex biological systems: Implications in health and disease

One of the metabolic processes that the holobiont should regulate and maintain in equilibrium is oxidoreduction (redox) (Wang, Oldham, Maron, & Loscalzo, 2018), this is of fundamental importance because the thermodynamic equilibrium of the microbiome is susceptible to being altered by an oxidative disruption that alters the microbial populations in interaction with the host (Million & Raoult, 2018). Thus, redox processes are regulated by the primary and secondary metabolism within the hologenome for cell development (DeLucia, Zavala, & Gog, 2018). In addition the hologenome to be shared due to the constant interaction of the holobiont is configured as an open genetic system (OGS) called symbiogenome and whose function is the structuring of the hologenome (Provorov, 2018). Thus, in the sharing of information in the microbiome host interactions, an equilibrium is established that predisposes or causes the disease (Simon et al., 2019). In this order of ideas, until now in this aspect of homeostasis of the holobiont, evidence has accumulated of its fundamental role in the neuro-immune-inflammatory axes (Kho & Lal, 2018). It has also been determined that the thermodynamic imbalance within the holobiont is evident in the alterations of the host microbiome, known as dysbiosis, a state that is associated with atopic diseases (Arrieta et al., 2018). So the interaction from birth with the eukaryotic microbiome will determine the cellular development and adaptive capacity of the human holobiont (Miller Jr., 2016). In addition, in dysbiosis, alterations of the secondary metabolites expressed in the BGCs are presented, suggesting changes in the hologenome coming from the imbalance of the molecular communication (Dorrestein, Mazmanian, & Knight, 2014).

On the other hand, not only the oxidative stress pathways in the dysbiosis are altered; this is how changes can also be observed in energy metabolism, defense mechanisms, and detoxification, as well as the absorption of nutrients (Gao et al., 2017). This is how the correct functionality of the symbiotic relationships that establish the sharing of information in the symbiogenome will determine a promising meta-Darwinian approach to the concept of health and disease (De Loof, 2017).

2.9 Biotechnological applications of hologenomics: The power of holobiontic adaptation

The hologenomic theory as a basis for achieving a balance of holobionts and ecosystems has been studied to be applied to improve sustainability in food production (Limborg et al., 2018); it is also considered capable of improving the functionality of the species and thus obtain varieties with greater fitness capacity and resistance to environmental changes (Nogales et al., 2015). Similarly, this potential of hologenomic and symbiogenomic evolution to treat human diseases related to inflammation and metabolic disorders is being explored (Singh, Ahmad, Musarrat, Ehtesham, & Hasnain, 2013) because it is considered a more effective way to keep the holobiont healthy and in homeostasis (McFall-Ngai et al., 2013). However, just as exciting will be the exploration of the chemical diversity coming from the different holobionts for the development of future medicines (van de Water, Allemand, & Ferrier-Pagès, 2018). This approach will also achieve a new pharmacology, capable of maintaining the networks of life that regulate thermodynamic equilibrium and homeostasis as a model of healing (Salvucci, 2016).

2.10 Conclusions

The search for thermodynamic equilibrium is the basis of survival and evolution of life, from its replication to its self-reference represented in cognition. In this attempt to share entropy, metabolic networks of molecular communicators have been established that regulate and exchange genetic information between and within the holobiont. Likewise, this interaction represented by the symbiogenome drives the change in the hologenome, causing the evolution of the holobiont as a whole. So, in this way, molecular communication modulates the homeostasis within the ecosystem and allows the adaptation of the individuals belonging to the niche. Equally, BGCs change and acquire new information to predict the environment and express the secondary metabolites needed to face the new challenges in order to regulate the metabolism to obtain energy from different sources. This delicate balance can be altered by oxidative stress, producing alteration of metabolic interactions inside the holobiont. In this way, oxidative disruption modifies microbial populations in exchange, inducing the appearance of the phenomenon of dysbiosis with the consequent implications for the health status of the biological system. Thus, the approximation of the theory of evolution based on the hologenome will be of fundamental importance in the development of a new model of health disease that allows the welfare of populations, as well as innovations for medicine and industry.

References

Aerts, J., Röling, W., Elsaesser, A., & Ehrenfreund, P. (2014). Biota and biomolecules in extreme environments on earth: Implications for life detection on Mars. *Life, 4*(4), 535–565.

Amedei, A., & Boem, F. (2018). I've gut a feeling: Microbiota impacting the conceptual and experimental perspectives of personalized medicine. *International Journal of Molecular Sciences, 19*(12), 3756.

Arrieta, M. C., Arévalo, A., Stiemsma, L., Dimitriu, P., Chico, M. E., Loor, S., … Turvey, S. E. (2018). Associations between infant fungal and bacterial dysbiosis and childhood atopic wheeze in a nonindustrialized setting. *Journal of Allergy and Clinical Immunology, 142*(2), 424–434.

Asplund-Samuelsson, J., Janasch, M., & Hudson, E. P. (2018). Thermodynamic analysis of computed pathways integrated into the metabolic networks of *E. coli* and *Synechocystis* reveals contrasting expansion potential. *Metabolic Engineering, 45*, 223–236.

Baedke, J. (2018). O organism, where art thou? Old and new challenges for organism-centered biology. *Journal of the History of Biology*, 1–32.

Bai, S., Ge, H., & Qian, H. (2018). Structure for energy cycle: A unique status of the second law of thermodynamics for living systems. *Science China Life Sciences, 61*(10), 1266–1273.

Bajić, D., Vila, J. C., Blount, Z. D., & Sánchez, A. (2018). On the deformability of an empirical fitness landscape by microbial evolution. *Proceedings of the National Academy of Sciences, 115*(44), 11286–11291.

Bapteste, E., & Huneman, P. (2018). Towards a dynamic interaction network of life to unify and expand the evolutionary theory. *BMC Biology, 16*(1), 56.

Baral, B., Akhgari, A., & Metsä-Ketelä, M. (2018). Activation of microbial secondary metabolic pathways: Avenues and challenges. *Synthetic and Systems Biotechnology, 3*(3), 163.

Basler, G., Fernie, A. R., & Nikoloski, Z. (2018). Advances in metabolic flux analysis toward genome-scale profiling of higher organisms. *Bioscience Reports, 38*(6), BSR20170224.

Baverstock, K. (2013). Life as physics and chemistry: A system view of biology. *Progress in Biophysics and Molecular Biology, 111*(2–3), 108–115.

Benavides-Mendoza, A. (2018). The terrestrial metasystem 2. *Energy, 1*, 34.

Brunetti, A. E., Neto, F. C., Vera, M. C., Taboada, C., Pavarini, D. P., Bauermeister, A., & Lopes, N. P. (2018). An integrative omics perspective for the analysis of chemical signals in ecological interactions. *Chemical Society Reviews, 47*(5), 1574–1591.

Carrier, T. J., & Reitzel, A. M. (2017). The hologenome across environments and the implications of a host-associated microbial repertoire. *Frontiers in Microbiology, 8*, 802.

Carthey, A. J., Gillings, M. R., & Blumstein, D. T. (2018). The extended genotype: Microbially mediated olfactory communication. *Trends in Ecology & Evolution, 33*(11), 885–894.

Catania, F., Krohs, U., Chittò, M., Ferro, D., Ferro, K., Lepennetier, G., … Gadau, J. (2017). The hologenome concept: We need to incorporate function. *Theory in Biosciences, 136*(3–4), 89–98.

Chen, B. S. (2018). *Systems evolutionary biology: Biological network evolution theory, stochastic evolutionary game strategies, and applications to systems synthetic biology*. Academic Press.

Cleary, J. L., Condren, A. R., Zink, K. E., & Sanchez, L. M. (2017). Calling all hosts: Bacterial communication in situ. *Chem, 2*(3), 334–358.

Colinas, M., & Goossens, A. (2018). Combinatorial transcriptional control of plant specialized metabolism. *Trends in Plant Science, 23*(4), 324–336.

Corning, P. A., & Szathmáry, E. (2015). "Synergistic selection": A Darwinian frame for the evolution of complexity. *Journal of Theoretical Biology, 371*, 45–58.

Corso-Díaz, X., Jaeger, C., Chaitankar, V., & Swaroop, A. (2018). Epigenetic control of gene regulation during development and disease: A view from the retina. *Progress in Retinal and Eye Research*.

Cruz-Morales, P., Kopp, J. F., Martínez-Guerrero, C., Yáñez-Guerra, L. A., Selem-Mojica, N., Ramos-Aboites, H., … Barona-Gomez, F. (2016). Phylogenomic analysis of natural products biosynthetic gene clusters allows discovery of arseno-organic metabolites in model streptomycetes. *Genome Biology and Evolution*, *8*(6), 1906–1916.

Dai, Z., & Locasale, J. W. (2018). Thermodynamic constraints on the regulation of metabolic fluxes. *Journal of Biological Chemistry*, *293*(51), 19725–19739.

Davies, P. C., Rieper, E., & Tuszynski, J. A. (2013). Self-organization and entropy reduction in a living cell. *Biosystems*, *111*(1), 1–10.

De Loof, A. (2017). The evolution of "life": A Metadarwinian integrative approach. *Communicative & Integrative Biology*, *10*(3), e1301335.

De Martino, D., Andersson, A. M., Bergmiller, T., Guet, C. C., & Tkačik, G. (2018). Statistical mechanics for metabolic networks during steady state growth. *Nature Communications*, *9*(1), 2988.

Del Carratore, F., Zych, K., Cummings, M., Takano, E., Medema, M., & Breitling, R. (2019). Computational identification of co-evolving multi-gene modules in microbial biosynthetic gene clusters. *Communications Biology*, *2*(83).

DeLucia, E. H., Zavala, J., & Gog, L. (2018). Linking primary and secondary metabolism a mechanistic hypothesis for how elevated CO_2 modulates defenses. In C. Emani (Ed.), *The biology of plant-insect interactions* (pp. 93–112). CRC Press.

Demetzos, C. (2015). Biophysics and thermodynamics: The scientific building blocks of bio-inspired drug delivery nano systems. *AAPS PharmSciTech*, *16*(3), 491–495.

Donia, M. S., Cimermancic, P., Schulze, C. J., Brown, L. C. W., Martin, J., Mitreva, M., … Fischbach, M. A. (2014). A systematic analysis of biosynthetic gene clusters in the human microbiome reveals a common family of antibiotics. *Cell*, *158*(6), 1402–1414.

Donohoe, D. R., & Bultman, S. J. (2012). Metaboloepigenetics: Interrelationships between energy metabolism and epigenetic control of gene expression. *Journal of Cellular Physiology*, *227*(9), 3169–3177.

Dorrestein, P. C., Mazmanian, S. K., & Knight, R. (2014). From microbiomess to metabolomes to function during host-microbial interactions. *Immunity*, *40*(6), 824.

Douglas, A. E. (2014). Symbiosis as a general principle in eukaryotic evolution. *Cold Spring Harbor Perspectives in Biology*, *6*(2), a016113.

Du, B., Zielinski, D. C., Monk, J. M., & Palsson, B. O. (2018). Thermodynamic favorability and pathway yield as evolutionary tradeoffs in biosynthetic pathway choice. *Proceedings of the National Academy of Sciences*, *115*(44), 11339–11344.

Duim, H., & Otto, S. (2017). Towards open-ended evolution in self-replicating molecular systems. *Beilstein Journal of Organic Chemistry*, *13*(1), 1189–1203.

Eckford, A. W., Kuznets-Speck, B., Hinczewski, M., & Thomas, P. J. (2018, June). *Thermodynamic properties of molecular communication*. In: *2018 IEEE international symposium on information theory (ISIT)*. IEEE. (pp. 2545–2549).

Epstein, O. (2018). The spatial homeostasis hypothesis. *Symmetry*, *10*(4), 103.

Femminella, M., Reali, G., & Vasilakos, A. V. (2015). A molecular communications model for drug delivery. *IEEE Transactions on Nanobioscience*, *14*(8), 935–945.

Fernandez-de-Cossio-Diaz, J., & Mulet, R. (2019). Maximum entropy and population heterogeneity in continuous cell cultures. *PLoS Computational Biology*, *15*(2), e1006823.

Gándara, L., & Wappner, P. (2018). Metabo-Devo: A metabolic perspective of development. *Mechanisms of Development*, *154*, 12–23.

Gao, B., Chi, L., Mahbub, R., Bian, X., Tu, P., Ru, H., & Lu, K. (2017). Multi-omics reveals that lead exposure disturbs gut microbiome development, key metabolites, and metabolic pathways. *Chemical Research in Toxicology*, *30*(4), 996–1005.

Gilbert, S. F., Bosch, T. C., & Ledón-Rettig, C. (2015). Eco-Evo-Devo: Developmental symbiosis and developmental plasticity as evolutionary agents. *Nature Reviews Genetics*, *16*(10), 611.

Hadacek, F., & Bachmann, G. (2015). Low-molecular-weight metabolite systems chemistry. *Frontiers in Environmental Science*, *3*, 12.

Hansen, L. D., Popovic, M., Tolley, H. D., & Woodfield, B. (2018). Laws of evolution parallel the laws of thermodynamics. *The Journal of Chemical Thermodynamics*, *124*, 141–148.

Harms, M. J., & Thornton, J. W. (2013). Evolutionary biochemistry: Revealing the historical and physical causes of protein properties. *Nature Reviews Genetics*, *14*(8), 559.

Hoogendoorn, K., Barra, L., Waalwijk, C., Dickschat, J. S., van der Lee, T., & Medema, M. H. (2018). Evolution and diversity of biosynthetic gene clusters in *Fusarium*. *Frontiers in Microbiology*, *9*, 1158.

Hurst, G. D. (2017). Extended genomes: Symbiosis and evolution. *Interface Focus*, *7*(5), 20170001.

Hutzil, S., Sandoval-Motta, S., Frank, A., & Aldana, M. (2018). Modeling the role of the microbiome in evolution. *Frontiers in Physiology*, *9*, 1836.

Kadloor, S., Adve, R. S., & Eckford, A. W. (2012). Molecular communication using brownian motion with drift. *IEEE Transactions on Nanobioscience*, *11*(2), 89–99.

Kaneko, K., & Furusawa, C. (2018). Macroscopic theory for evolving biological systems akin to thermodynamics. *Annual Review of Biophysics*, *47*, 273–290.

Keller, N. P. (2018). Fungal secondary metabolism: Regulation, function and drug discovery. *Nature Reviews Microbiology*, *1*, .

Keller, L., & Surette, M. G. (2006). Communication in bacteria: An ecological and evolutionary perspective. *Nature Reviews Microbiology*, *4*(4), 249.

Kessler, A., & Kalske, A. (2018). Plant secondary metabolite diversity and species interactions. *Annual Review of Ecology, Evolution, and Systematics*, *49*, 115–138.

Kho, Z. Y., & Lal, S. K. (2018). The human gut microbiome—A potential controller of wellness and disease. *Frontiers in Microbiology*, *9*, .

Kirchhoff, M., Parr, T., Palacios, E., Friston, K., & Kiverstein, J. (2018). The Markov blankets of life: Autonomy, active inference and the free energy principle. *Journal of the Royal Society Interface*, *15*(138), 20170792.

Koch, L. G., & Britton, S. L. (2018). Evolutionary origin of disease and complexity: A non-equilibrium thermodynamic solution. *bioRxiv*, 356493.

Kompanichenko, V. (2014). Emergence of biological organization through thermodynamic inversion. *Frontiers in Bioscience (Elite Edition)*, *6*, 208–224.

Kong, W., Meldgin, D. R., Collins, J. J., & Lu, T. (2018). Designing microbial consortia with defined social interactions. *Nature Chemical Biology*, *14*(8), 821.

Kutschera, U. (2018). Systems biology of eukaryotic superorganisms and the holobiont concept. *Theory in Biosciences*, *137*(2), 117–131.

Lambert, J. P., Picaud, S., Fujisawa, T., Hou, H., Savitsky, P., Uusküla-Reimand, L., … Knight, J. D. (2019). Interactome rewiring following pharmacological targeting of BET bromodomains. *Molecular Cell*, *73*(3), 621–638.

Lancet, D., Zidovetzki, R., & Markovitch, O. (2018). Systems protobiology: Origin of life in lipid catalytic networks. *Journal of the Royal Society Interface*, *15*(144), 20180159.

Last, C. (2015). Human metasystem transition (HMST) theory. *Journal of Evolution and Technology*, *25*(1), 1–16.

Li, X. H., Chavali, P. L., Pancsa, R., Chavali, S., & Babu, M. M. (2018). Function and regulation of phase-separated biological condensates. *Biochemistry*, *57*(17), 2452–2461.

Li, X., & Snyder, M. (2011). Metabolites as global regulators: A new view of protein regulation: Systematic investigation of metabolite-protein interactions may help bridge the gap between genome-wide association studies and small molecule screening studies. *BioEssays*, *33*(7), 485–489.

Limborg, M. T., Alberdi, A., Kodama, M., Roggenbuck, M., Kristiansen, K., & Gilbert, M. T. P. (2018). Applied hologenomics: Feasibility and potential in aquaculture. *Trends in Biotechnology*, *36*(3), 252–264.

Liu, T., Ma, C. J., Yuan, B. F., & Feng, Y. Q. (2018). Modificaomics: Deciphering the functions of biomolecule modifications. *Science China Chemistry*, 1–12.

Lyon, P. (2007). From quorum to cooperation: Lessons from bacterial sociality for evolutionary theory. *Studies in History and Philosophy of Science Part C: Studies in History and Philosophy of Biological and Biomedical Sciences*, *38*(4), 820–833.

Maity, B. K., Vishvakarma, V., Surendran, D., Rawat, A., Das, A., Pramanik, S., … Maiti, S. (2018). Spontaneous fluctuations can guide drug design strategies for structurally disordered proteins. *Biochemistry*, *57*(28), 4206–4213.

McFall-Ngai, M., Hadfield, M. G., Bosch, T. C., Carey, H. V., Domazet-Lošo, T., Douglas, A. E., … Hentschel, U. (2013). Animals in a bacterial world, a new imperative for the life sciences. *Proceedings of the National Academy of Sciences*, *110*(9), 3229–3236.

Meier, J. L. (2013). Metabolic mechanisms of epigenetic regulation. *ACS Chemical Biology*, *8*(12), 2607–2621.

Mendoza, M. L. Z., Xiong, Z., Escalera-Zamudio, M., Runge, A. K., Thézé, J., Streicker, D., … Castruita, J. A. S. (2018). Hologenomic adaptations underlying the evolution of sanguivory in the common vampire bat. *Nature Ecology & Evolution*, *2*(4), 659.

Metallo, C. M., & Vander Heiden, M. G. (2010). Metabolism strikes back: Metabolic flux regulates cell signaling. *Genes & Development*, *24*(24), 2717–2722.

Metallo, C. M., & Vander Heiden, M. G. (2013). Understanding metabolic regulation and its influence on cell physiology. *Molecular Cell*, *49*(3), 388–398.

Miller, W. (2016). Cognition, information fields and hologenomic entanglement: Evolution in light and shadow. *Biology*, *5*(2), 21.

Miller, W. B., Jr. (2016). The eukaryotic microbiome: Origins and implications for fetal and neonatal life. *Frontiers in Pediatrics*, *4*, 96.

Miller, W. B., Jr. (2018). Biological information systems: Evolution as cognition-based information management. *Progress in Biophysics and Molecular Biology*, *134*, 1–26.

Miller, W. B., Jr., & Torday, J. S. (2018). Four domains: The fundamental unicell and post-Darwinian cognition-based evolution. *Progress in Biophysics and Molecular Biology*, *140*, 49–73.

Miller, W. B., Jr., Torday, J. S., & Baluška, F. (2018). Biological evolution as defense of 'self'. *Progress in Biophysics and Molecular Biology*.

Million, M., & Raoult, D. (2018). Linking gut redox to human microbiome. *Human Microbiome Journal*, *10*, 27–32.

Miyazawa, H., & Aulehla, A. (2018). Revisiting the role of metabolism during development. *Development*, *145*(19), dev131110.

Moral, R. D., González, M., Navarro, J., & Marijuán, P. C. (2011). From genomics to scientomics: Expanding the bioinformation paradigm. *Information*, *2*(4), 651–671.

Moran, N. A., & Sloan, D. B. (2015). The hologenome concept: Helpful or hollow? *PLoS Biology*, *13*(12), e1002311.

Morris, J. J. (2018). What is the hologenome concept of evolution? *F1000Research*, 7, .

Mossio, M., & Bich, L. (2017). What makes biological organisation teleological? *Synthese*, *194*(4), 1089–1114.

Muraille, E. (2018). Diversity generator mechanisms are essential components of biological systems: The two queen hypothesis. *Frontiers in Microbiology*, *9*, 223.

Naviaux, R. K. (2018). Metabolic features and regulation of the healing cycle-A new model for chronic disease pathogenesis and treatment. *Mitochondrion*.

Nee, S. (2016). The evolutionary ecology of molecular replicators. *Royal Society Open Science*, *3*(8), 160235.

Noda-Garcia, L., Liebermeister, W., & Tawfik, D. S. (2018). Metabolite–enzyme coevolution: From single enzymes to metabolic pathways and networks. *Annual Review of Biochemistry*, *87*, 187–216.

Nogales, A., Nobre, T., Valadas, V., Ragonezi, C., Döring, M., Polidoros, A., & Arnholdt-Schmitt, B. (2015). Can functional hologenomics aid tackling current challenges in plant breeding? *Briefings in Functional Genomics*, *15*(4), 288–297.

Okada, B. K., & Seyedsayamdost, M. R. (2017). Antibiotic dialogues: Induction of silent biosynthetic gene clusters by exogenous small molecules. *FEMS Microbiology Reviews*, *41*(1), 19–33.

Pasinetti, G. M., Singh, R., Westfall, S., Herman, F., Faith, J., & Ho, L. (2018). The role of the gut microbiota in the metabolism of polyphenols as characterized by gnotobiotic mice. *Journal of Alzheimer's Disease*, 1–13. [preprint].

Patra, B., Schluttenhofer, C., Wu, Y., Pattanaik, S., & Yuan, L. (2013). Transcriptional regulation of secondary metabolite biosynthesis in plants. *Biochimica et Biophysica Acta (BBA)-Gene Regulatory Mechanisms*, *1829*(11), 1236–1247.

Pereira, A., Vimal, R. L. P., & Pregnolato, M. (2017). *Can qualitative biophysics solve the hard problem?* In *Biophysics of consciousness: A foundational approach*. Singapore: World Scientific Publishing. (pp. 149–188).

Petrakis, S., & Andrade-Navarro, M. A. (2016). Protein interaction networks in health and disease. *Frontiers in Genetics*, 7, 111.

Piazza, I., Kochanowski, K., Cappelletti, V., Fuhrer, T., Noor, E., Sauer, U., & Picotti, P. (2018). A map of protein-metabolite interactions reveals principles of chemical communication. *Cell*, *172*(1–2), 358–372.

Piñero, J., & Solé, R. (2018). Nonequilibrium entropic bounds for Darwinian replicators. *Entropy*, *20*(2), 98.

Pinu, F. R., Granucci, N., Daniell, J., Han, T. L., Carneiro, S., Rocha, I., … Villas-Boas, S. G. (2018). Metabolite secretion in microorganisms: The theory of metabolic overflow put to the test. *Metabolomics*, *14*(4), 43.

Planqué, R., Hulshof, J., Teusink, B., Hendriks, J. C., & Bruggeman, F. J. (2018). Maintaining maximal metabolic flux by gene expression control. *PLoS Computational Biology*, *14*(9), e1006412.

Porcar, M. (2019). The hidden charm of life. *Life*, *9*(1), 5.

Pross, A. (2004). Causation and the origin of life. Metabolism or replication first? *Origins of Life and Evolution of the Biosphere*, *34*(3), 307–321.

Pross, A. (2005). On the chemical nature and origin of teleonomy. *Origins of Life and Evolution of Biospheres*, *35*(4), 383–394.

Provorov, N. A. (2018). Symbiogenesis as evolution of open genetic systems. *Russian Journal of Genetics*, *54*(8), 888–896.

Raes, J., & Bork, P. (2008). Molecular eco-systems biology: Towards an understanding of community function. *Nature Reviews Microbiology*, *6*(9), 693.

Reen, F. J., McGlacken, G. P., & O'Gara, F. (2018). The expanding horizon of alkyl quinolone signalling and communication in polycellular interactomes. *FEMS Microbiology Letters*, *365*(9), fny076.

Reynés, B., Palou, M., Rodríguez, A. M., & Palou, A. (2019). Regulation of adaptive thermogenesis and browning by prebiotics and postbiotics. *Frontiers in Physiology*, *9*, 1908.

Rigali, S., Anderssen, S., Naômé, A., & van Wezel, G. P. (2018). Cracking the regulatory code of biosynthetic gene clusters as a strategy for natural product discovery. *Biochemical Pharmacology*, *153*, 24–34.

Rosenberg, E., Sharon, G., Atad, I., & Zilber-Rosenberg, I. (2010). The evolution of animals and plants via symbiosis with microorganisms. *Environmental Microbiology Reports*, *2*(4), 500–506.

Rosenberg, E., & Zilber-Rosenberg, I. (2018). The hologenome concept of evolution after 10 years. *Microbiome*, *6*(1), 78.

Rosenberg, E., & Zilber-Rosenberg, I. (2019). The Hologenome concept of evolution: Medical implications. *Rambam Maimonides Medical Journal*, *10*(1).

Roughgarden, J., Gilbert, S. F., Rosenberg, E., Zilber-Rosenberg, I., & Lloyd, E. A. (2018). Holobionts as units of selection and a model of their population dynamics and evolution. *Biological Theory, 13*(1), 44–65.

Salvucci, E. (2016). Microbiome, holobiont and the net of life. *Critical Reviews in Microbiology, 42*(3), 485–494.

Schlitter, J. (2018). The second law of thermodynamics as a force law. *Entropy, 20*(4), 234.

Seoane, L. F., & Solé, R.V. (2018). Information theory, predictability and the emergence of complex life. *Royal Society Open Science, 5*(2), 172221.

Sharon, G., Garg, N., Debelius, J., Knight, R., Dorrestein, P. C., & Mazmanian, S. K. (2014). Specialized metabolites from the microbiome in health and disease. *Cell Metabolism, 20*(5), 719–730.

Simon, J. C., Marchesi, J. R., Mougel, C., & Selosse, M. A. (2019). Host-microbiota interactions: From holobiont theory to analysis. *Microbiome*, 7(1), 5.

Singh, Y., Ahmad, J., Musarrat, J., Ehtesham, N. Z., & Hasnain, S. E. (2013). Emerging importance of holobionts in evolution and in probiotics. *Gut pathogens, 5*(1), 12.

Sinumvayo, J. P., Zhao, C., & Tuyishime, P. (2018). Recent advances and future trends of riboswitches: Attractive regulatory tools. *World Journal of Microbiology and Biotechnology, 34*(11), 171.

Sitaraman, R. (2018). Prokaryotic horizontal gene transfer within the human holobiont: Ecological-evolutionary inferences, implications and possibilities. *Microbiome, 6*(1), 163.

Skene, K. (2015). Life's a gas: A thermodynamic theory of biological evolution. *Entropy, 17*(8), 5522–5548.

Smith, R. L., Soeters, M. R., Wüst, R. C., & Houtkooper, R. H. (2018). Metabolic flexibility as an adaptation to energy resources and requirements in health and disease. *Endocrine Reviews, 39*(4), 489–517.

Speed, M. P., Fenton, A., Jones, M. G., Ruxton, G. D., & Brockhurst, M.A. (2015). Coevolution can explain defensive secondary metabolite diversity in plants. *New Phytologist, 208*(4), 1251–1263.

Tarabichi, M., Antoniou, A., Saiselet, M., Pita, J. M., Andry, G., Dumont, J. E., … Maenhaut, C. (2013). Systems biology of cancer: Entropy, disorder, and selection-driven evolution to independence, invasion and "swarm intelligence". *Cancer and Metastasis Reviews, 32*(3–4), 403–421.

Tessera, M. (2018). Is pre-Darwinian evolution plausible? *Biology Direct, 13*(1), 18.

Torday, J. S., Miller, W. B., Jr. (2017). The resolution of ambiguity as the basis for life: A cellular bridge between Western reductionism and Eastern holism. *Progress in Biophysics and Molecular Biology, 131*, 288–297.

Torday, J. S., Miller, W. B., Jr. (2018). Terminal addition in a cellular world. *Progress in Biophysics and Molecular Biology, 135*, 1–10.

Trosko, J. (2016). Evolution of microbial quorum sensing to human global quorum sensing: An insight into how gap junctional intercellular communication might be linked to the global metabolic disease crisis. *Biology, 5*(2), 29.

Tsuruyama, T. (2018). The conservation of average entropy production rate in a model of signal transduction: Information thermodynamics based on the fluctuation theorem. *Entropy, 20*(4), 303.

Tu, Y., & Rappel, W. J. (2018). Adaptation in living systems. *Annual review of condensed matter physics, 9*, 183–205.

van de Water, J. A., Allemand, D., & Ferrier-Pagès, C. (2018). Host-microbe interactions in octocoral holobionts-recent advances and perspectives. *Microbiome, 6*(1), 64.

Vitas, M., & Dobovišek, A. (2018). In the beginning was a mutualism—On the origin of translation. *Origins of Life and Evolution of Biospheres, 48*, 223–243.

Voss, J. D., Leon, J. C., Dhurandhar, N.V., & Robb, F.T. (2015). Pawnobiome: Manipulation of the hologenome within one host generation and beyond. *Frontiers in Microbiology, 6*, 697.

Wang, R. S., Oldham, W. M., Maron, B. A., & Loscalzo, J. (2018). Systems biology approaches to redox metabolism in stress and disease states. *Antioxidants & Redox Signaling, 29*(10), 953–972.

Yan, Q., Lopes, L. D., Shaffer, B. T., Kidarsa, T. A., Vining, O., Philmus, B., … Andreote, F. D. (2018). Secondary metabolism and interspecific competition affect accumulation of spontaneous mutants in the GacS-GacA regulatory system in *Pseudomonas protegens. mBio, 9*(1), e01845-17.

Zhao, Q. (2013). Nature of protein dynamics and thermodynamics. *Reviews in Theoretical Science, 1*(1), 83–101.

Zivieri, R., & Pacini, N. (2018). Entropy density acceleration and minimum dissipation principle: Correlation with heat and matter transfer in glucose catabolism. *Entropy, 20*(12), 929.

zu Castell, W., Lüttge, U., & Matyssek, R. (2019). Gaia—A holobiont-like system emerging from interaction. In L. Wegner & L. Ulrich (Eds.), *Emergence and modularity in life sciences* (pp. 255–279). Cham: Springer.

CHAPTER 3

Natural products and molecular networks

There is little doubt that the planetary patina—including ourselves—is autopoietic. Life at the surface of the Earth seems to regulate itself in the face of external perturbation, and does so without regard for the individuals and species that compose it. More than 99.99 percent of the species that have ever existed have become extinct, but the planetary patina, with its army of cells, have continued for more than three billion years. … trillions of communicating, evolving microbes. The visible world is a late-arriving, overgrown portion of the microcosm, and it functions only because of its well-developed connection with the microcosm's activities.

Natural selection eliminates and maybe maintains, but it doesn't create… Neo-Darwinists say that new species emerge when mutations occur and modify an organism. I was taught over and over again that the accumulation of random mutations led to evolutionary change [which] led to new species. I believed it until I looked for evidence.

Lynn Margulis (1938–2011)

3.1 Introduction

Natural products (NPs) are defined as the chemical substances produced by the secondary metabolism of living organisms; in this way, the secondary metabolites are those that regulate the interaction of the biological system with the environment (Seyedsayamdost, 2019). Likewise, NPs help regulate the primary metabolism to optimize the acquisition of nutrients with which to maintain cellular functionality (Barreiro & Martínez-Castro, 2019). Equally, metabolites function as growth factor signaling that controls the nutrient acquisition and cellular proliferation to maintain system homeostasis (Björklund, 2019). In addition, NPs can control the transport of the same nutrients through downregulation mechanisms (Fig. 1) (Savir, Martynov, & Springer, 2017), which makes the secondary metabolites key

Molecular Evolutionary Models in Drug Discovery
https://doi.org/10.1016/B978-0-12-817613-9.00003-1

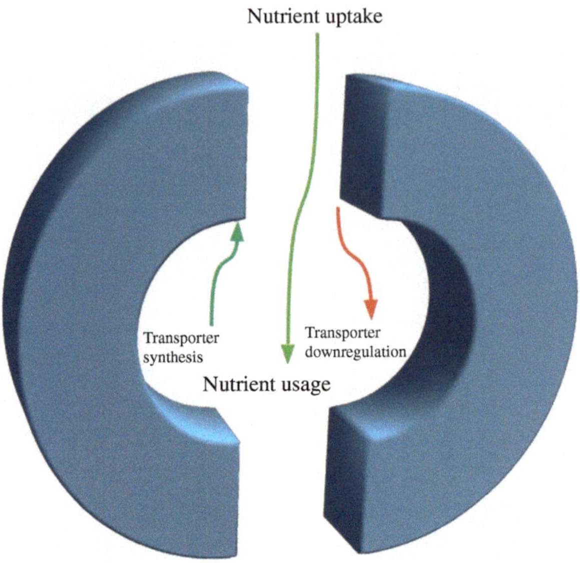

Fig. 1 Homeostasis in nutrients uptake.

players in the maintenance of metabolic homeostasis and the sharing of entropy (Fernandez-de-Cossio-Diaz & Vazquez, 2018). Likewise, the presence of groups of biosynthetic genes (BCG) in cells demonstrates their evolution through chemical defense pathways, which act as molecular communication within the biological system (Olsen & Small, 2018). On the other hand, both prokaryotic and eukaryotic organisms have developed systems to establish signal transport communication networks of secondary metabolites, where extracellular membrane vesicles are highlighted (Hoefler et al., 2017; Yáñez-Mó et al., 2015). In this way, it is considered that these compounds and their transport mechanisms originated in order to establish molecular networks of interaction (Deveau et al., 2018; Lyu, Hu, Fu, & Xing, 2018). Thus the configuration of networks gives dynamism, diversity and complexity to the system; that is why the metabolic pathways, both primary and secondary, complement each other for the acquisition of fitness (Fig. 2) (Green et al., 2018).

This is how these energy networks and metabolic interactions allow collaboration between holobionts in the metasystem and lead to complex adaptations being made (Embree, Liu, Al-Bassam, & Zengler, 2015; Pál & Papp, 2017). In addition, these multispecies consortia are in constant coevolution between macrobes and microbiota, which is demonstrated in the chemical diversity and complexity of their molecular

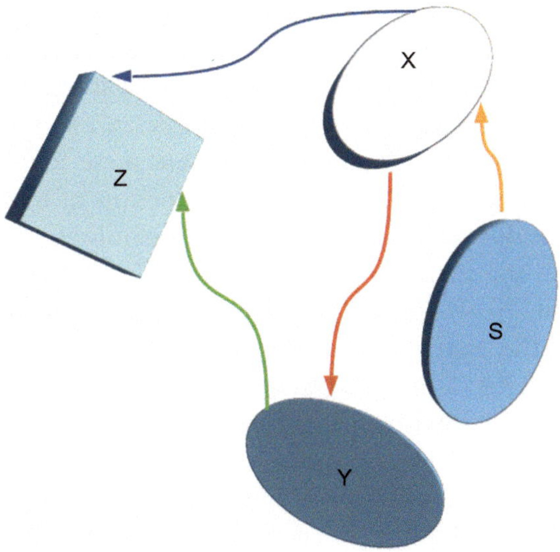

Fig. 2 Molecular network model.

communicators (Bourrat & Griffiths, 2018). Likewise, secondary metabolites can activate the epigenetic control of the transcription of specific genes in order to carry out various adaptive functions within the cell (Cichewicz, 2010). These epigenetic regulators from secondary metabolism (e.g., curcumin, resveratrol, and genistein) have shown their activity in diseases such as cancer by performing a homeostatic control on alterations of the primary metabolism that underlie this condition (Mirza, Shah, Patel, Jain, & Rawal, 2018). Equally, this epigenetic control is exercised over the signaling systems, in order to balance the biological systems affected (Miceli, Bontempo, Nebbioso, & Altucci, 2014; Ratovitski, 2017). Therefore, the objective of this chapter is to explore the functionality of the NPs for the establishment of cellular communication networks and their role in the acquisition of the thermodynamic equilibrium necessary for the holobiont's evolution.

3.2 Life and secondary metabolism: Interactions in evolution

The secondary metabolites are key pieces in the interaction of the organisms with their environment; these are synthesized by proteins encoded in the BGCs, which regulate their chemical diversity (Krause et al., 2018; Wilson, Zha, & Balskus, 2017). So, these mediators of mutual support facilitate coevolution regulating growth, cell behavior, and self-reference (Stachowicz, 2001); they are also the molecular communicators of the symbiosis in the holobiont (Švorcová, Markoš, & Das, 2018), in what is considered a microcosm of metabolic signals that allow persistence and survival, as has been demonstrated in microbial communities, where these multispecies associations employ antibiotics as signaling and induction of biofilm formation (Shank, 2018). In the same way, in eukaryotic organisms, there is a delicate balance between the metabolism and the signaling system in mutual regulation (Laxman, 2017). In addition, the secondary metabolism has been fundamental in the appearance of the molecular replicators that allowed the development from a prebiotic to a biotic phase in the origin of life on Earth, due to the ecological and evolutionary stability that these provide (Szilágyi et al., 2017).

Thus the establishment of metabolic networks becomes fundamental in the coevolution that allows the acquisition of fitness being key for the evolution of prebiotic RNA (Copley, Smith, & Morowitz, 2007; Pande & Kost, 2017). This evolution was also made possible due to the action of metabolic enzymes that became specialized as the catalyzed processes granted greater adaptive capacity (Juárez-Vázquez et al., 2017; Peracchi, 2018), as well as by the recruitment of enzymes that confer selective advantage to the host as they are affected by random genetic mutations that permit acquiring new catalytic functions (Schulenburg & Miller, 2014). Continuing in this sense, the expansion of several genes that encode the same enzymatic functions managed to obtain a robustness of the primary metabolism that finally achieved a stability of secondary metabolism in environmental changes such as the limitation of nutrients (Schniete et al., 2018). In addition, is important take into account that this robustness depends on the ecological adaptations and the lifestyle of the species—for example, high robustness is observed in fast growers and reflects higher production of secondary metabolites, as has been observed in bacteria (Freilich et al., 2010)—although the robustness of genetic systems is also present in eukaryotes as a source of diversity (Payne & Wagner, 2018). Thus, the global vision of secondary metabolism connects us to diverse processes that have a functionality within the biological system, and which allow the primary metabolism to optimize the obtaining of energy; this approach leads us to elucidate the role of the NPs in the evolution and diversity of species by allowing communication and exchange with the environment (Carrington et al., 2018; Wink, 2018).

3.3 Natural products as molecular communicators

NPs are the core of the biotic interaction, where they act as messenger molecules for the benefit of the cells that produce them (Meinwald, 2010). Thus, in the conformation of signal networks that interact constantly, biological systems acquire cognition and ability to predict, anticipate, learn to solve problems and create self-reference (Lyon, 2015). Likewise, the establishment of molecular communication networks leads to the self-organization of biological systems, as observed in the complex adaptive systems (CAS) that make up the bacteria through quorum sensing-mediated signaling (Fig. 3) (Cunha, Xavier, & de Castro, 2018). In this order of ideas, these chemical signals can maintain the homeostasis of the developing system and induce the expression of new spatial patterns of genes that can lead to changes and phenotypic adaptations (Nijhout, Best, & Reed, 2018). It is also important to note that when developing intercellular interactions it is possible to increase the negative entropy of the system by giving it a thermodynamic equilibrium, which is why chemical communication is the basis to maintain the evolutionary dynamic (Brändas, 2018).

On the other hand, this capacity for self-organization is energized by the transmission of information to the interior of the system, which allows the development of sensors, transporters, signaling cascades, and transcription factors (Larsen et al., 2018; Rosas, Mediano, Ugarte, & Jensen, 2018); that is, the cells transmit information within the network using

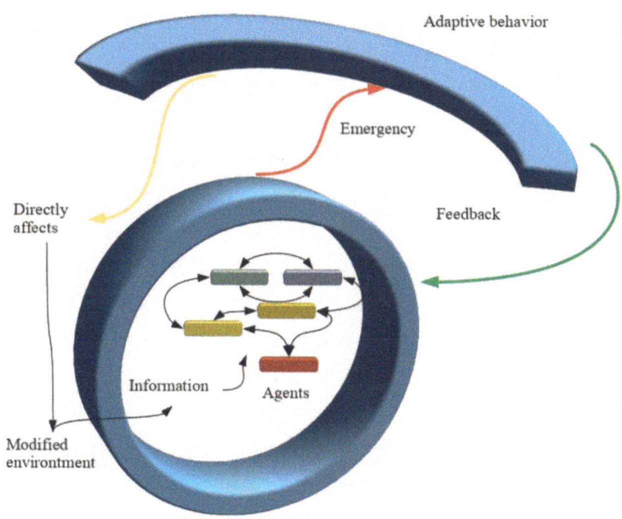

Fig. 3 Processing of information in complex adaptive systems (CAS).

secondary metabolites in order to establish an association in the biological system (Jahagirdar, Suarez-Diez, & Saccenti, 2019). Likewise, this signal transduction network is integrated with the genome-scale metabolic network and transcriptional regulatory network (Hao et al., 2018), which leads to a metabolic organization that becomes autocatalytic and dynamic through communication mediated by molecular messengers. In this way, this integration of genetic information with signal transduction evolved in bacteria through adaptations mediated by ribozymes, whose regulation is carried out through their metabolite sensors or riboswitches (Serganov & Patel, 2007, 2012). This is what makes this evolutionary factor a promising molecular tool in the investigation of secondary metabolites from bacteria (Machtel et al., 2016). This is how we are dealing with a chemical communication system coming from a RNA world and which is also regulated by the ability to interact and read information about the environment, as the wide chemical diversity has evolved through communication, interaction, and survival (Chatterjee & Yadav, 2019).

3.4 Natural products: Networks in the RNA world

The hypothesis of an RNA world proposes the passage from an abiotic to a biotic world through RNA as the self-replicating molecule capable of storing information, performing protein synthesis, and catalytic functions (Lancet, Zidovetzki, & Markovitch, 2018; Neveu, Kim, & Benner, 2013). Logically the theories of first RNA or first metabolism are not in apparent contradiction—they are mostly complementary—because it was necessary that the existence of spontaneous chemical reactions capable of developing energetic processes so that a ribonucleopeptide could be self-sustaining (Danchin, 2017). So the next tendencies will be more directed toward a theory integrated in the functionality of the processes based on complex networks, but not to the identification of a single moment of the origin of life. This is because it is there, in the application of concepts, where the function envisages that cooperative associations arise when integrating chemical processes with the capacity to perform an information management to establish much more sophisticated metabolic processes (Stewart, 2014).

In this way, the application of secondary metabolism in remnants of the RNA world such as ribozymes and riboswitches has been key to the development of innovative medicines such as streptomycin (Disney, Dwyer, & Childs-Disney, 2018). The interaction of small molecules with RNA explains how molecular signaling in microorganisms is carried out with a communication established by the secondary metabolites; additionally, this interaction regulates the synthesis of other metabolites by the recipient cell (Piazza et al., 2018). Then, under this antibiotic dialogue, the gene expression is induced, the chemical diversity is encouraged, and fitness acquired (Okada & Seyedsayamdost, 2017). Thus, this evolution induced by antibiotics in the field of competition and cooperation can achieve the homeostasis of the biological system within the holobiont (Bauer, Kainz, Carmona-Gutierrez, & Madeo, 2018; Ponziani et al., 2016).

3.5 Epigenetics of secondary metabolism

As the network formed by the RNA world and metabolic systems acquires its complexity to the extent that it can predict environmental changes and can cooperate with other organisms, so the secondary metabolism takes another connotation to be regulated in an evolutionary way by the epigenome (Farnsworth, Albantakis, & Caruso, 2017; Strauss & Reyes-Dominguez, 2011). In this way, the BGCs are regulated in their transcription by environmental stimuli and depend on the state of development of the organism; also, the nutritional state induces or represses the synthesis of secondary metabolites (Keller, 2018). Thus, in eukaryotes, chromatin remodeling through methylation and acetylation of histones is one of the most common epigenetic mechanisms of regulation of biosynthetic genes (Baral, Akhgari, & Metsä-Ketelä, 2018). Likewise, the secondary metabolites produced may have the ability to induce chromatin-modifying enzymes, which helps maintain metabolic states in homeostasis (Nieborak & Schneider, 2018). In addition, these epigenetic modifications obey a phenotypic adaptive response to the environment and chemical signals emitted by other organisms of the biological system; similarly, they lead to persistent changes of genotypic type, where we can observe again the role of molecular communicators in evolution (Burggren, 2016). Moreover, this network of chemical signals that induce epigenetic modifications also represents another factor of cognition, self-reference, and self-organization of the biological systems belonging to a metasystem (Day & Sweatt, 2011; Schneider-Poetsch & Yoshida, 2018). Thus, the epigenetic regulation takes a role in the maintenance of a thermodynamic equilibrium and a decrease in entropy, which maintains the metabolic dynamics (Boccardi, Comanducci, Baroni, & Mecocci, 2017). This also confers a fundamental factor of metabolism secondary to the healing cycle as a bioenergetic and metabolic balance (Naviaux, 2018). Additionally, this pharmacological potential of natural products on the epigenetic regulation of metabolic equilibrium will be promising in the search for new therapeutic alternatives (Remely et al., 2015).

3.6 The symbiotic holobiont as a molecular network

So a holobiont is established in a balance that allows it to evolve through the metabolic networks that are woven between the microbiome and the host (Richardson, 2017). By forming an evolutionary unit, the holobiont not only enters a dialectic of coevolution, it also exchanges information among all the individuals that make it up and makes molecular communications with the environment and other holobionts (Chiu & Gilbert, 2015). Likewise, in this constant exchange of molecular signals, the holobiont undergoes changes in its hologenome that lead it to obtain greater adaptive capacity (Schnorr, Sankaranarayanan, Lewis Jr., & Warinner, 2016). In this way, secondary metabolites are produced by the host in response to quorum sensing signals from microbiome; this exchange of information will derive in epigenetic modifications of gene expression on both sides (Fig. 4) (Turroni, Brigidi, Cavalli, & Candela, 2017). Additionally, it is important to take into consideration the exchange that the microbiome makes with the environment surrounding the host and the capacity of the microorganisms to transduce environmental signals and communicate them to the

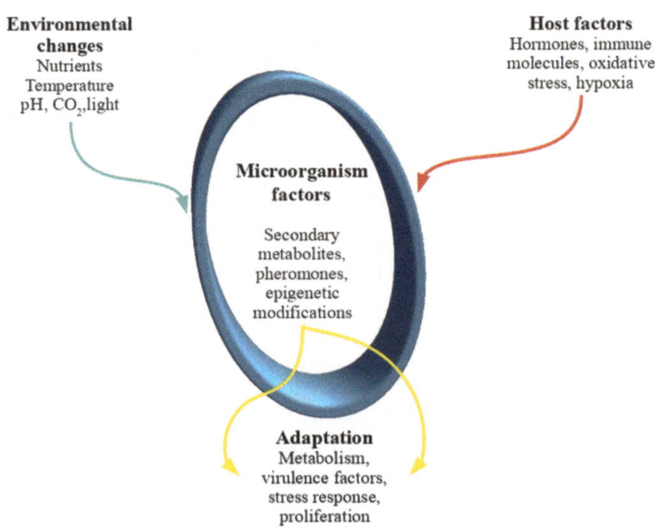

Fig. 4 Microbiome sensing of environmental changes.

interior of the holobiont (Braunsdorf, Mailänder-Sánchez, & Schaller, 2016; Koskella, Hall, & Metcalf, 2017). In this way, chemical signals are produced by virtue of environmental changes and induce an adaptive response within the biological system when transduced from the microbiome to the host (Slijepcevic, 2018). In addition, this communication network in constant balance can be interrupted by intense exposure to environmental factors such as antibiotics and diet, as seen in inflammation and cancer (Lewis et al., 2015; Yang et al., 2018). Furthermore, this disruption of molecular communication causes the production of secondary metabolites that lead to a failure of the symbiosis (Lamont & Hajishengallis, 2015; Mazzocca, Ferraro, Misciagna, & Fais, 2018). In this way, the failure of the symbiosis or dysbiosis alters the metabolism of the microbiome and consequently the information received by the host with the consequent erratic response of the same (Lajczak, Mroz, Saint-Criq, & Keely, 2016; Larsen & Dai, 2015). Likewise, the search for new therapeutic alternatives that seek to reverse microbial dysbiosis will be a promising field of action in the integral treatment of both acute and chronic diseases (Gregor, David, & Meijler, 2018; Zheng et al., 2018).

3.7 Chemical signaling and the hologenome

Now, after all of the above, it is important to ask: does molecular signaling change the hologenome, and if so, what could be the metabolic pathways through which it takes place? Of course, it is already a fact that symbionts alter the genetics of the host and that the acquisition of microbial genes is a fundamental evolutionary factor in the complexity of biological systems (Rosenberg & Zilber-Rosenberg, 2016). In this way, the products of secondary metabolism favor adaptation and genetic exchange between the symbionts and the host (Adam et al., 2018). This chemical ecology of hologenome supports the formation of chemical networks that facilitate the exchange and genetic transfer that allows the acquisition of fitness by the host (Pita, Rix, Slaby, Franke, & Hentschel, 2018). Thus, the molecular communications of the microbiome in response to environmental factors induce changes in the hologenome that lead to the evolution and diversity of the species, as has been determined in the influence of the response of the microbiome and its evolution against dietary changes (van de Guchte, Blottière, & Doré, 2018).

Equally, in this transkingdom network the production of small molecules regulates gene expression, allowing physiological homeostasis to be reached (Davison et al., 2017; Meisel et al., 2018). On the other hand, the pharmacological implications of the intervention with drugs must be taken into account in this delicate balance. This is a topic that has gained strength due to the study of the physiological and toxic events that may occur under a new branch known as pharmacomicrobiomics, where medicines are already a new environmental factor that can induce changes in the holobiont (Doestzada et al., 2018; Panebianco, Andriulli, & Pazienza, 2018). In addition, the recovery of microbiome ecosystem using prebiotics, probiotics, and synbiotics, as well as fecal microbiota transplantation (FMT) and bacterial consortium transplantation (BCT) can open the gates to new functionalities of the microbiome both from the metabolic and genetic point of view (Adak & Khan, 2019; Gagliardi et al., 2018). Equally, new frontiers in human development as a holobiont in constant interaction can be projected and evaluated (Dominguez-Bello, Godoy-Vitorino, Knight, & Blaser, 2019).

3.8 Holobiont health communication and symbiosis

The metabolic disruption of the symbiosis and its reconstruction will become a new paradigm of health (Postler & Ghosh, 2017) in which the restoration of the microbiome and its metabolic interactions within the holobiont will be studied, as well as its evolutionary implications (Limborg & Heeb, 2018; Raina et al., 2018). Additionally, in these ecological restoration processes, the chemical defenses presented by the symbionts and the host's immune response should be integrated (Orr, Kocurek, & Young, 2018), as well as control over the environmental factors in which the restoration of the microbiome will be carried out, to allow the restoration of the thermodynamic equilibrium of the biological system (Bauer & Thiele, 2018; Sen & Orešič, 2019). Thus, the use of prebiotics, probiotics, and synbiotics for re-establishment of the holobiont symbiosis network could be a novel field in antimicrobial therapy, as well as a new adjuvant strategy in the management of metabolic diseases and cancer (Markowiak & Śliżewska, 2017, 2018).

However, in this way it will be necessary to recognize the role of the virome in microbiota and host homeostasis within the holobiont (Grasis, 2017). Likewise, the role of the mycobioma in the balance of the microbiome will be another factor to be determined, because it has been shown to be altered during disease, which suggests its regulatory potential (Cui, Morris, & Ghedin, 2013). So in this way it has been possible to establish a connection between viroma and mycobioma as well as bacteriophages in disorders of glucose metabolism (Stefanaki, Peppa, Mastorakos, & Chrousos, 2017). For this reason, an integral approach to the restoration of the microbiome must be conceived from the molecular signaling of a multibiome; that is, from an ecosystemic vision (Filyk & Osborne, 2016). Likewise, evaluating the metabolomics of the multibiome could elucidate the role of secondary metabolites as molecular communicators and inducers of adaptation and fitness acquisition (Blacher, Levy, Tatirovsky, & Elinav, 2017). Additionally, the effects of the metabolites produced (hormones, proteins, and small molecules) by the host microbiota interaction on the hologenome must be determined to reduce the risk of inflammation, cancer, and autoimmune disorders (Benbow, Pechal, Tomberlin, & Jordan, 2018). On the other hand, another interesting approach is the use of small molecules to modulate the chemical signals between the host and its symbionts in order to achieve eubiosis (Beebe, Sampey, Watkins, Milburn, & Eckhart, 2014; Adnani, Rajski, & Bugni, 2017). Finally, the hologenomic approach, in which the health of the holobiont can be maintained through the control of gene expression or repression that regulates interaction and communication, is an exciting field in the discovery of new drugs, but it is necessary to increase our understanding of the ecological associations involved (Miller, Svanbäck, & Bohannan, 2018; Theis, 2018).

3.9 Conclusions

The establishment of molecular signal networks within biological systems makes secondary metabolism crucial in the search for stability and optimization of the use of energy sources. In this way, NPs as bioactive molecules exert an effector function that allows regulating through chemical communication the acquisition of fitness in a given ecosystem (Craney, Ozimok, Pimentel-Elardo, Capretta, & Nodwell, 2012). This is how metabolic networks allow the exchange between the symbionts and the host that make up the holobionts (Esser et al., 2018); this intercommunication will lead to the adaptation of the holobiont as a whole to environmental changes and later to its evolution (Stencel & Wloch-Salamon, 2018). In this way, the pharmacological modulation of the symbiotic interactions of the holobiont is a promising field in medicine because of its impacts for the treatment of infectious diseases and cancer, as well as metabolic disorders (Malla et al., 2018). This novel approach seeks to restore the balance in the intercommunications between host and symbionts, as well as their relations of commensalism and mutualism (Garcia & Gerardo, 2014). It has also been shown that chemically diverse molecules produced by the secondary metabolism (genistein, lycopene, resveratrol, curcumin, and pectin) have activity on therapeutic targets capable of modulating the microbiota and their interactions with the host (Greiner, Papineni, & Umar, 2014), which already speaks to us now about the future use of prebiotics, probiotics, and synbiotics as chemopreventive medicines for use in clinical practice (Thilakarathna, Langille, & Rupasinghe, 2018). Finally, to develop pharmacological agents that regulate gene expression and protein production in different organs and tissues, with what we could already modulate the molecular communication networks for the maintenance of a healthy holobiont (Lee, Song, Nam, & Lee, 2018), requires an ecosystemic vision of living beings as complex biological units that interact in a metasystem where they adapt as they share information (Ryan, Jones, Hayes, & Craig, 2019).

References

Adak, A., & Khan, M. R. (2019). An insight into gut microbiota and its functionalities. *Cellular and Molecular Life Sciences*, *76*, 473–493.

Adam, Z. R., Kacar, B., Som, S. M., Lynch, K. L., Walther-Antonio, M., & Williford, K. H. (2018). The origin of animals as microbial host volumes in nutrient-limited seas. *PeerJ Preprints*, *6*, e27173v1.

Adnani, N., Rajski, S. R., & Bugni, T. S. (2017). Symbiosis-inspired approaches to antibiotic discovery. *Natural Product Reports*, *34*(7), 784–814.

Baral, B., Akhgari, A., & Metsä-Ketelä, M. (2018). Activation of microbial secondary metabolic pathways: Avenues and challenges. *Synthetic and Systems Biotechnology*, *3*(3), 163.

Barreiro, C., & Martínez-Castro, M. (2019). Regulation of the phosphate metabolism in Streptomyces genus: Impact on the secondary metabolites. *Applied Microbiology and Biotechnology*, 1–16.

Bauer, M. A., Kainz, K., Carmona-Gutierrez, D., & Madeo, F. (2018). Microbial wars: Competition in ecological niches and within the microbiome. *Microbial Cell*, *5*(5), 215.

Bauer, E., & Thiele, I. (2018). From network analysis to functional metabolic modeling of the human gut microbiota. *mSystems*, *3*(3), e00209-17.

Beebe, K., Sampey, B., Watkins, S. M., Milburn, M., & Eckhart, A. D. (2014). Understanding the apothecaries within: The necessity of a systematic approach for defining the chemical output of the human microbiome. *Clinical and Translational Science*, 7(1), 74–81.

Benbow, M. E., Pechal, J. L., Tomberlin, J. K., & Jordan, H. R. (2018). Interkingdom community interactions in disease ecology. In C. J. Hurst (Ed.), *The connections between ecology and infectious disease* (pp. 3–38). Cham: Springer.

Björklund, M. (2019). Cell size homeostasis: Metabolic control of growth and cell division. *Biochimica et Biophysica Acta (BBA)-Molecular Cell Research*, *1866*(3), 409–417.

Blacher, E., Levy, M., Tatirovsky, E., & Elinav, E. (2017). Microbiome-modulated metabolites at the interface of host immunity. *The Journal of Immunology*, *198*(2), 572–580.

Boccardi, V., Comanducci, C., Baroni, M., & Mecocci, P. (2017). Of energy and entropy: The ineluctable impact of aging in old age dementia. *International Journal of Molecular Sciences*, *18*(12), 2672.

Bourrat, P., & Griffiths, P. E. (2018). Multispecies individuals. *History and Philosophy of the Life Sciences*, *40*(2), 33.

Brändas, E. J. (2018). A simple communication hypothesis: The process of evolution reconsidered. In E. J. Brändas (Ed.), *Concepts, methods and applications of quantum systems in chemistry and physics* (pp. 381–404). Cham: Springer.

Braunsdorf, C., Mailänder-Sánchez, D., & Schaller, M. (2016). Fungal sensing of host environment. *Cellular Microbiology*, *18*(9), 1188–1200.

Burggren, W. (2016). Epigenetic inheritance and its role in evolutionary biology: Re-evaluation and new perspectives. *Biology*, *5*(2), 24.

Carrington, Y., Guo, J., Le, C. H., Fillo, A., Kwon, J., Tran, L. T., & Ehlting, J. (2018). Evolution of a secondary metabolic pathway from primary metabolism: Shikimate and quinate biosynthesis in plants. *The Plant Journal*, *95*(5), 823–833.

Chatterjee, S., & Yadav, S. (2019). The origin of prebiotic information system in the peptide/RNA world: A simulation model of the evolution of translation and the genetic code. *Life*, *9*(1), 25.

Chiu, L., & Gilbert, S. F. (2015). The birth of the holobiont: Multi-species birthing through mutual scaffolding and niche construction. *Biosemiotics*, *8*(2), 191–210.

Cichewicz, R. H. (2010). Epigenome manipulation as a pathway to new natural product scaffolds and their congeners. *Natural Product Reports*, *27*(1), 11–22.

Copley, S. D., Smith, E., & Morowitz, H. J. (2007). The origin of the RNA world: Co-evolution of genes and metabolism. *Bioorganic Chemistry*, *35*(6), 430–443.

Craney, A., Ozimok, C., Pimentel-Elardo, S. M., Capretta, A., & Nodwell, J. R. (2012). Chemical perturbation of secondary metabolism demonstrates important links to primary metabolism. *Chemistry & Biology*, *19*(8), 1020–1027.

Cui, L., Morris, A., & Ghedin, E. (2013). The human mycobiome in health and disease. *Genome Medicine*, *5*(7), 63.

Cunha, D., Xavier, R., & de Castro, L. N. (2018). Bacterial colonies as complex adaptive systems. *Natural Computing*, *17*(4), 781–798.

Danchin, A. (2017). From chemical metabolism to life: The origin of the genetic coding process. *Beilstein Journal of Organic Chemistry*, *13*(1), 1119–1135.

Davison, J. M., Lickwar, C. R., Song, L., Breton, G., Crawford, G. E., & Rawls, J. F. (2017). Microbiota regulate intestinal epithelial gene expression by suppressing the transcription factor hepatocyte nuclear factor 4 alpha. *Genome Research*, *27*(7), 1195–1206.

Day, J. J., & Sweatt, J. D. (2011). Epigenetic mechanisms in cognition. *Neuron*, *70*(5), 813–829.

Deveau, A., Bonito, G., Uehling, J., Paoletti, M., Becker, M., Bindschedler, S., … Mieszkin, S. (2018). Bacterial–fungal interactions: Ecology, mechanisms and challenges. *FEMS Microbiology Reviews*, *42*(3), 335–352.

Disney, M. D., Dwyer, B. G., & Childs-Disney, J. L. (2018). Drugging the RNA world. *Cold Spring Harbor Perspectives in Biology*, *10*(11), a034769.

Doestzada, M., Vila, A. V., Zhernakova, A., Koonen, D. P., Weersma, R. K., Touw, D. J., … Fu, J. (2018). Pharmacomicrobiomics: A novel route toward personalized medicine? *Protein & Cell*, *9*, 432–445.

Dominguez-Bello, M. G., Godoy-Vitorino, F., Knight, R., & Blaser, M. J. (2019). Role of the microbiome in human development. *Gut*, *68*(6), 1108–1114.

Embree, M., Liu, J. K., Al-Bassam, M. M., & Zengler, K. (2015). Networks of energetic and metabolic interactions define dynamics in microbial communities. *Proceedings of the National Academy of Sciences*, *112*(50), 15450–15455.

Esser, D., Lange, J., Marinos, G., Sieber, M., Best, L., Prasse, D., … Sommer, F. (2018). Functions of the microbiota for the physiology of animal Metaorganisms. *Journal of Innate Immunity*, 1–12.

Farnsworth, K. D., Albantakis, L., & Caruso, T. (2017). Unifying concepts of biological function from molecules to ecosystems. *Oikos*, *126*(10), 1367–1376.

Fernandez-de-Cossio-Diaz, J., & Vazquez, A. (2018). A physical model of cell metabolism. *Scientific Reports*, *8*(1), 8349.

Filyk, H. A., & Osborne, L. C. (2016). The multibiome: The intestinal ecosystem's influence on immune homeostasis, health, and disease. *eBioMedicine*, *13*, 46–54.

Freilich, S., Kreimer, A., Borenstein, E., Gophna, U., Sharan, R., & Ruppin, E. (2010). Decoupling environment-dependent and independent genetic robustness across bacterial species. *PLoS Computational Biology*, *6*(2), e1000690.

Gagliardi, A., Totino, V., Cacciotti, F., Iebba, V., Neroni, B., Bonfiglio, G., ... Schippa, S. (2018). Rebuilding the gut microbiota ecosystem. *International Journal of Environmental Research and Public Health*, *15*(8), 1679.

Garcia, J. R., & Gerardo, N. M. (2014). The symbiont side of symbiosis: Do microbes really benefit? *Frontiers in Microbiology*, *5*, 510.

Grasis, J. A. (2017). The intra-dependence of viruses and the holobiont. *Frontiers in Immunology*, *8*, 1501.

Green, S., Şerban, M., Scholl, R., Jones, N., Brigandt, I., & Bechtel, W. (2018). Network analyses in systems biology: New strategies for dealing with biological complexity. *Synthese*, *195*(4), 1751–1777.

Gregor, R., David, S., & Meijler, M. M. (2018). Chemical strategies to unravel bacterial–eukaryotic signaling. *Chemical Society Reviews*, *47*(5), 1761–1772.

Greiner, A. K., Papineni, R. V., & Umar, S. (2014). Chemoprevention in gastrointestinal physiology and disease. Natural products and microbiome. *American Journal of Physiology Gastrointestinal and Liver Physiology*, *307*, G1–G15.

Hao, T., Wu, D., Zhao, L., Wang, Q., Wang, E., & Sun, J. (2018). The genome-scale integrated networks in microorganisms. *Frontiers in Microbiology*, *9*, 296.

Hoefler, B. C., Stubbendieck, R. M., Josyula, N. K., Moisan, S. M., Schulze, E. M., & Straight, P. D. (2017). A link between linearmycin biosynthesis and extracellular vesicle genesis connects specialized metabolism and bacterial membrane physiology. *Cell Chemical Biology*, *24*(10), 1238–1249.

Jahagirdar, S., Suarez-Diez, M., & Saccenti, E. (2019). Simulation and reconstruction of metabolite-metabolite association networks using a metabolic dynamic model and correlation based-algorithms. *Journal of Proteome Research*, *18*(3), 1099–1113.

Juárez-Vázquez, A. L., Edirisinghe, J. N., Verduzco-Castro, E. A., Michalska, K., Wu, C., Noda-García, L., ... Carrillo-Tripp, M. (2017). Evolution of substrate specificity in a retained enzyme driven by gene loss. *eLife*, *6*, e22679.

Keller, N. P. (2018). Fungal secondary metabolism: Regulation, function and drug discovery. *Nature Reviews Microbiology*, *1*, .

Koskella, B., Hall, L. J., & Metcalf, C. J. E. (2017). The microbiome beyond the horizon of ecological and evolutionary theory. *Nature Ecology & Evolution*, *1*(11), 1606.

Krause, D. J., Kominek, J., Opulente, D. A., Shen, X. X., Zhou, X., Langdon, Q. K., ... Hittinger, C.T. (2018). Functional and evolutionary characterization of a secondary metabolite gene cluster in budding yeasts. *Proceedings of the National Academy of Sciences*, *115*(43), 11030–11035.

Lajczak, N. K., Mroz, M. S., Saint-Criq, V., & Keely, S. (2016). Bile acids regulate intestinal epithelial restitution: Implications for pathogenesis and therapy of IBD. *The FASEB Journal*, *30*(1 Suppl), 1023–1028.

Lamont, R. J., & Hajishengallis, G. (2015). Polymicrobial synergy and dysbiosis in inflammatory disease. *Trends in Molecular Medicine*, *21*(3), 172–183.

Lancet, D., Zidovetzki, R., & Markovitch, O. (2018). Systems protobiology: Origin of life in lipid catalytic networks. *Journal of the Royal Society Interface*, *15*(144), 20180159.

Larsen, P. E., & Dai, Y. (2015). Metabolome of human gut microbiome is predictive of host dysbiosis. *Gigascience*, *4*(1), 42.

Larsen, P. E., Zerbs, S., Laible, P. D., Collart, F. R., Korajczyk, P., Dai, Y., & Noirot, P. (2018). Modeling the Pseudomonas sulfur regulome by quantifying the storage and communication of information. *mSystems*, *3*(3), e00189-17.

Laxman, S. (2017). Conceptualizing eukaryotic metabolic sensing and signaling. *Journal of the Indian Institute of Science*, *97*(1), 59–77.

Lee, E. S., Song, E. J., Nam, Y. D., & Lee, S.Y. (2018). Probiotics in human health and disease: From nutribiotics to pharmabiotics. *Journal of Microbiology*, *56*(11), 773–782.

Lewis, J. D., Chen, E. Z., Baldassano, R. N., Otley, A. R., Griffiths, A. M., Lee, D., ... Albenberg, L. (2015). Inflammation, antibiotics, and diet as environmental stressors of the gut microbiome in pediatric Crohn's disease. *Cell Host & Microbe*, *18*(4), 489–500.

Limborg, M. T., & Heeb, P. (2018). Coevolution of hosts and their microbiome. *Genes*, *9*(11).

Lyon, P. (2015). The cognitive cell: Bacterial behavior reconsidered. *Frontiers in Microbiology*, *6*, 264.

Lyu, L., Hu, M., Fu, A., & Xing, B. (2018). Extracellular vesicle directed exogenous ion channel transport for precise manipulation of biological events. *Bioconjugate Chemistry*, *29*(8), 2715–2722.

Machtel, P., Bąkowska-Żywicka, K., & Żywicki, M. (2016). Emerging applications of riboswitches–from antibacterial targets to molecular tools. *Journal of applied genetics*, *57*(4), 531–541.

Malla, M. A., Dubey, A., Kumar, A., Yadav, S., Hashem, A., & Abd_Allah, E. F. (2018). Exploring the human microbiome: The potential future role of next-generation sequencing in disease diagnosis and treatment. *Frontiers in Immunology*, *9*, .

Markowiak, P., & Śliżewska, K. (2017). Effects of probiotics, prebiotics, and synbiotics on human health. *Nutrients*, *9*(9), 1021.

Markowiak, P., & Śliżewska, K. (2018). The role of probiotics, prebiotics and synbiotics in animal nutrition. *Gut Pathogens*, *10*(1), 21.

Mazzocca, A., Ferraro, G., Misciagna, G., & Fais, S. (2018). Moving the systemic evolutionary approach to cancer forward: Therapeutic implications. *Medical Hypotheses*, *121*, 80–87.

Meinwald, J. (2010). Natural products as molecular messengers. *Journal of Natural Products*, *74*(3), 305–309.

Meisel, J. S., Sfyroera, G., Bartow-McKenney, C., Gimblet, C., Bugayev, J., Horwinski, J., ... Hodkinson, B. P. (2018). Commensal microbiota modulate gene expression in the skin. *Microbiome*, *6*(1), 20.

Miceli, M., Bontempo, P., Nebbioso, A., & Altucci, L. (2014). Natural compounds in epigenetics: A current view. *Food and Chemical Toxicology*, *73*, 71–83.

Miller, E. T., Svanbäck, R., & Bohannan, B. J. (2018). Microbiomes as metacommunities: Understanding host-associated microbes through metacommunity ecology. *Trends in Ecology & Evolution*, *33*(12), 926–935.

Mirza, S., Shah, K., Patel, S., Jain, N., & Rawal, R. (2018). Natural compounds as epigenetic regulators of human dendritic cell-mediated immune function. *Journal of Immunotherapy*, *41*(4), 169–180.

Naviaux, R. K. (2018). Metabolic features and regulation of the healing cycle—A new model for chronic disease pathogenesis and treatment. *Mitochondrion*, . pii: S1567-7249(18)30105-3.

Neveu, M., Kim, H. J., & Benner, S. A. (2013). The "strong" RNA world hypothesis: Fifty years old. *Astrobiology*, *13*(4), 391–403.

Nieborak, A., & Schneider, R. (2018). Metabolic intermediates–Cellular messengers talking to chromatin modifiers. *Molecular metabolism*, *14*, 39–52.

Nijhout, H. F., Best, J. A., & Reed, M. C. (2018). Systems biology of robustness and homeostatic mechanisms. *Wiley Interdisciplinary Reviews: Systems Biology and Medicine*, e1440.

Okada, B. K., & Seyedsayamdost, M. R. (2017). Antibiotic dialogues: Induction of silent biosynthetic gene clusters by exogenous small molecules. *FEMS Microbiology Reviews*, *41*(1), 19–33.

Olsen, K. M., & Small, L. L. (2018). Micro-and macroevolutionary adaptation through repeated loss of a complete metabolic pathway. *New Phytologist, 219*(2), 757–766.
Orr, M. R., Kocurek, K. M., & Young, D. L. (2018). Gut microbiota and human health: Insights from ecological restoration. *The Quarterly Review of Biology, 93*(2), 73–90.
Pál, C., & Papp, B. (2017). Evolution of complex adaptations in molecular systems. *Nature Ecology & Evolution, 1*(8), 1084.
Pande, S., & Kost, C. (2017). Bacterial unculturability and the formation of intercellular metabolic networks. *Trends in Microbiology, 25*(5), 349–361.
Panebianco, C., Andriulli, A., & Pazienza, V. (2018). Pharmacomicrobiomics: Exploiting the drug-microbiota interactions in anticancer therapies. *Microbiome, 6*(1), 92.
Payne, J. L., & Wagner, A. (2018). The causes of evolvability and their evolution. *Nature Reviews Genetics, 1*, .
Peracchi, A. (2018). The limits of enzyme specificity and the evolution of metabolism. *Trends in Biochemical Sciences, 43*(12), 984–996.
Piazza, I., Kochanowski, K., Cappelletti, V., Fuhrer, T., Noor, E., Sauer, U., & Picotti, P. (2018). A map of protein-metabolite interactions reveals principles of chemical communication. *Cell, 172*(1–2), 358–372.
Pita, L., Rix, L., Slaby, B. M., Franke, A., & Hentschel, U. (2018). The sponge holobiont in a changing ocean: From microbes to ecosystems. *Microbiome, 6*(1), 46.
Ponziani, F. R., Scaldaferri, F., Petito, V., Sterbini, F. P., Pecere, S., Lopetuso, L. R., … Cammarota, G. (2016). The role of antibiotics in gut microbiota modulation: The eubiotic effects of rifaximin. *Digestive Diseases, 34*(3), 269–278.
Postler, T. S., & Ghosh, S. (2017). Understanding the holobiont: How microbial metabolites affect human health and shape the immune system. *Cell Metabolism, 26*(1), 110–130.
Raina, J. B., Eme, L., Pollock, F. J., Spang, A., Archibald, J. M., & Williams, T. A. (2018). Symbiosis in the microbial world: From ecology to genome evolution. *Biology Open*, 7(2), bio032524.
Ratovitski, E. A. (2017). Anticancer natural compounds as epigenetic modulators of gene expression. *Current Genomics, 18*(2), 175–205.
Remely, M., Lovrecic, L., Garza, A. L., Migliore, L., Peterlin, B., Milagro, F. I., … Haslberger, A. G. (2015). Therapeutic perspectives of epigenetically active nutrients. *British Journal of Pharmacology, 172*(11), 2756–2768.
Richardson, L. A. (2017). Evolving as a holobiont. *PLoS Biology, 15*(2), e2002168.
Rosas, F., Mediano, P., Ugarte, M., & Jensen, H. (2018). An information-theoretic approach to self-organisation: Emergence of complex interdependencies in coupled dynamical systems. *Entropy, 20*(10), 793.
Rosenberg, E., & Zilber-Rosenberg, I. (2016). Microbes drive evolution of animals and plants: The hologenome concept. *MBio*, 7(2), e01395-15.
Ryan, J. T., Jones, S., Hayes, P. A., & Craig, J. M. (2019). Leadership evolution for planetary health: A genomics perspective. *Challenges, 10*(1), 4.
Savir, Y., Martynov, A., & Springer, M. (2017). Achieving global perfect homeostasis through transporter regulation. *PLoS Computational Biology, 13*(4), e1005458.
Schneider-Poetsch, T., & Yoshida, M. (2018). Along the central dogma—Controlling gene expression with small molecules. *Annual Review of Biochemistry, 87*, 391–420.
Schniete, J. K., Cruz-Morales, P., Selem-Mojica, N., Fernández-Martínez, L. T., Hunter, I. S., Barona-Gómez, F., & Hoskisson, P. A. (2018). Expanding primary metabolism helps generate the metabolic robustness to facilitate antibiotic biosynthesis in streptomyces. *MBio, 9*(1), e02283-17.
Schnorr, S. L., Sankaranarayanan, K., Lewis, C. M., Jr., & Warinner, C. (2016). Insights into human evolution from ancient and contemporary microbiome studies. *Current Opinion in Genetics & Development, 41*, 14–26.
Schulenburg, C., & Miller, B. G. (2014). Enzyme recruitment and its role in metabolic expansion. *Biochemistry, 53*(5), 836–845.

Sen, P., & Orešič, M. (2019). Metabolic modeling of human gut microbiota on a genome scale: An overview. *Metabolites*, *9*(2), 22.

Serganov, A., & Patel, D. J. (2007). Ribozymes, riboswitches and beyond: Regulation of gene expression without proteins. *Nature Reviews Genetics*, *8*(10), 776.

Serganov, A., & Patel, D. J. (2012). Metabolite recognition principles and molecular mechanisms underlying riboswitch function. *Annual Review of Biophysics*, *41*, 343–370.

Seyedsayamdost, M. R. (2019). Toward a global picture of bacterial secondary metabolism. *Journal of Industrial Microbiology & Biotechnology*, 1–11.

Shank, E. A. (2018). Considering the lives of microbes in microbial communities. *mSystems*, *3*(2), e00155-17.

Slijepcevic, P. (2018). Evolutionary epistemology: Reviewing and reviving with new data the research programme for distributed biological intelligence. *Biosystems*, *163*, 23–35.

Stachowicz, J. J. (2001). Mutualism, facilitation, and the structure of ecological communities: Positive interactions play a critical, but underappreciated, role in ecological communities by reducing physical or biotic stresses in existing habitats and by creating new habitats on which many species depend. *Bioscience*, *51*(3), 235–246.

Stefanaki, C., Peppa, M., Mastorakos, G., & Chrousos, G. P. (2017). Examining the gut bacteriome, virome, and mycobiome in glucose metabolism disorders: Are we on the right track? *Metabolism*, *73*, 52–66.

Stencel, A., & Wloch-Salamon, D. M. (2018). Some theoretical insights into the hologenome theory of evolution and the role of microbes in speciation. *Theory in Biosciences*, *137*(2), 197–206.

Stewart, J. E. (2014). The direction of evolution: The rise of cooperative organization. *Biosystems*, *123*, 27–36.

Strauss, J., & Reyes-Dominguez, Y. (2011). Regulation of secondary metabolism by chromatin structure and epigenetic codes. *Fungal Genetics and Biology*, *48*(1), 62–69.

Švorcová, J., Markoš, A., & Das, P. (2018). Origins of the cellular biosphere. In V. P. Sahi & F. Baluska (Eds.), *Concepts in cell biology-history and evolution* (pp. 271–290). Cham: Springer.

Szilágyi, A., Zachar, I., Scheuring, I., Kun, Á., Könnyű, B., & Czárán, T. (2017). Ecology and evolution in the RNA world dynamics and stability of prebiotic replicator systems. *Life*, *7*(4), 48.

Theis, K. R. (2018). Hologenomics: Systems-level host biology. *mSystems*, *3*, e00164-17.

Thilakarathna, W. W., Langille, M. G., & Rupasinghe, H. V. (2018). Polyphenol-based prebiotics and synbiotics: Potential for cancer chemoprevention. *Current Opinion in Food Science*, *20*, 51–57.

Turroni, S., Brigidi, P., Cavalli, A., & Candela, M. (2017). Microbiota–host transgenomic metabolism, bioactive molecules from the inside: Miniperspective. *Journal of Medicinal Chemistry*, *61*(1), 47–61.

van de Guchte, M., Blottière, H. M., & Doré, J. (2018). Humans as holobionts: Implications for prevention and therapy. *Microbiome*, *6*(1), 81.

Wilson, M. R., Zha, L., & Balskus, E. P. (2017). Natural product discovery from the human microbiome. *Journal of Biological Chemistry*, *292*(21), 8546–8552.

Wink, M. (2018). Introduction: Biochemistry, physiology and ecological functions of secondary metabolites. *Annual Plant Reviews Online*, 1–19.

Yáñez-Mó, M., Siljander, P. R. M., Andreu, Z., Bedina Zavec, A., Borràs, F. E., Buzas, E. I., … Colás, E. (2015). Biological properties of extracellular vesicles and their physiological functions. *Journal of extracellular vesicles*, *4*(1), 27066.

Yang, X., Da, M., Zhang, W., Qi, Q., Zhang, C., & Han, S. (2018). Role of *Lactobacillus* in cervical cancer. *Cancer Management and Research*, *10*, 1219.

Zheng, J., Yuan, X., Cheng, G., Jiao, S., Feng, C., Zhao, X., … Liu, H. (2018). Chitosan oligosaccharides improve the disturbance in glucose metabolism and reverse the dysbiosis of gut microbiota in diabetic mice. *Carbohydrate Polymers*, *190*, 77–86.

Further reading

Engl, T., Kroiss, J., Kai, M., Nechitaylo, T.Y., Svatoš, A., & Kaltenpoth, M. (2018). Evolutionary stability of antibiotic protection in a defensive symbiosis. *Proceedings of the National Academy of Sciences, 115*(9), E2020–E2029.

Rosenberg, E. (2016). Collective memory and the hologenome concept. *Global Journal of Medical Research, 16*(3), 17–23.

Schvartzman, J. M., Thompson, C. B., & Finley, L. W. (2018). Metabolic regulation of chromatin modifications and gene expression. *The Journal of Cell Biology, 217*(7), 2247–2259.

CHAPTER 4

Chemical evolution: Life as the lab of the universe

Living matter evades the decay to equilibrium

if we were organisms so sensitive that a single atom, or even a few atoms, could make a perceptible impression on our senses – Heavens, what would life be like! To stress one point: an organism of that kind would most certainly not be capable of developing the kind of orderly thought which, after passing through a long sequence of earlier stages, ultimately results in forming, among many other ideas, the idea of an atom.

Erwin Schrödinger (1887–1961)

So how can we test the idea that the transition from nonlife to life is simple enough to happen repeatedly? The most obvious and straightforward way is to search for a second form of life on Earth. No planet is more Earth-like than Earth itself, so if the path to life is easy, then life should have started up many times over right here.

Paul Davies (1946–)

4.1 Introduction

The chemical evolution of the secondary metabolites shows us the common origin of the biosynthetic pathways, as well as the biological functions exerted by these chemically diverse molecules (Beran, Köllner, Gershenzon, & Tholl, 2019; Chezem & Clay, 2016). In this way, the secondary metabolites were initially components of the primary metabolism that later acquired specialized functions in chemical defense and molecular signaling; an example are the families of terpenes that are common to many metabolic pathways as well as to many kinds of species (bacteria, fungi, and amoebae between them) (Chen et al., 2016). In addition, this type of molecule evolved from the ecological interactions between the biotic and abiotic

Molecular Evolutionary Models in Drug Discovery
https://doi.org/10.1016/B978-0-12-817613-9.00004-3

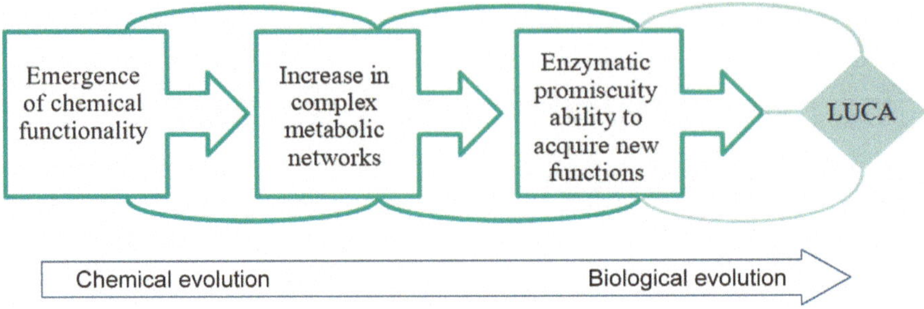

Fig. 1 Chemical to biological evolution transition.

aspects of the environment that surrounded the living beings that produced them (Lange, 2015; Pichersky & Raguso, 2018). In addition, these biotic interactions have allowed the evolution of functionality in biological systems from the underlying chemical reactions, also acquiring autonomy to establish exchange networks that will configure an ecosystem (Fig. 1) (Ruiz-Mirazo, Briones, & de la Escosura, 2017).

So, independent replicators are associated in signaling networks that have the ability to innovate as a means of survival (Solé, 2016). In this way, the abiotic synthesis of the molecules of life (amino acids, peptides, ribose, nucleic acids, fatty acids, and nucleotides) required specific environmental conditions of reaction (gas phase, pH, temperature, and dry and wet cycles, among others) to achieve the necessary biological functions that allowed them to manage their metabolism and regulate it (Kitadai & Maruyama, 2018). Likewise, the biotic interactions sustained by the biological activity of chemical evolution made it possible to adapt to environmental changes and acquire fitness, enhancing the diversity of life (Brodie et al., 2017; Lawrence et al., 2012). Similarly, the functionality in chemical evolution is acquired in communication with other complex biological systems, so that the primary metabolism passed to the secondary metabolism to achieve regulation and optimization in the processes of use of energy (Szappanos et al., 2016). These innovations in molecular evolution are achieved by accumulating highly specific mutations that bring benefits to the living system (Wilke, 2012). For this reason, enzymes and their adaptations as innovation mechanisms played an important role in this aspect (Arnold, 2018a, 2018b).

So in this way, the metabolic dynamics of the protocells was developed by the ribozymes modeling the first metabolic networks in their process and kinetics (Pechuan, Puzio, & Bergman, 2018). Equally, the presence of alarmones, in all species that are ribonucleotide derivatives synthesized under stress conditions, are widely distributed in nature (e.g., cAMP). They are considered to be ancient molecules that combine catalytic functions with genetic information that are a result of the evolution of molecular signaling from the RNA world, which connects us to the beginning of the biotic world with the last universal common ancestor or LUCA (Hernández-Morales, Becerra, & Lazcano, 2019). Interestingly, these alarmones continue to be indispensable in microorganisms like secondary messengers that perform a sensory function of the environment for adaptation (Hauryliuk, Atkinson, Murakami, Tenson, & Gerdes, 2015); as is the case of bis-(3′,5′)-cyclic diguanosine monophosphate (c-di-GMP), which is crucial for the adhesion and induction of biofilms—one of the oldest adaptation mechanisms of bacteria (Hengge et al., 2019). All this seems to confirm that these messenger nucleotides are the first chemical signals of the RNA world from which the current communication networks with which the biological systems acquired complexity were established (Nelson & Breaker, 2017). Finally, this opens the possibility to consider that the current natural products (NPs) as a result of secondary metabolism can act as a substrate or inhibitor of the nucleotide second messengers to exert their pharmacological action (Abusnina & Lugnier, 2017).

Therefore, the objective of this chapter is to establish the connection between chemical and biological evolution from the RNA world to complex biological systems as a model of innovation in the development of new therapeutic alternatives.

4.2 Chemical evolution and communication in the RNA world

Cellular life requires the RNA network for DNA replication, this network is made up of rRNA, tRNA, and mRNA (ribosomal, transfer, and messenger). The functions of this network allow communication with other systems to remain in coevolution (Villarreal & Witzany, 2019). This RNA world determined the origin of life on Earth and evolved from a prebiotic stage where there were protonucleotides that were formed from chemical reactions under terrestrial environmental conditions (Hud, 2018). In this way, the RNA acquired self-replicating and cooperative capacity to regulate the necessary metabolic processes using the chemical reactions present (Higgs & Lehman, 2015; O'Flaherty et al., 2018). Thus, life could go from a thermodynamic self-assembly to a kinetic auto-assembly thanks to molecular intercommunications that the RNA network established for the management of the metabolic processes (Pross & Pascal, 2017). In addition, these self-assembly systems were a fundamental part for the establishment of the physiological functions necessary for life to become self-sustaining (Wang, Liu, Xing, & Yan, 2016).

In this way, due to the tendency shown by organisms to self-organization, each autonomous organization could be grouped into biological systems where chemical evolution managed to develop diverse structures capable of sharing information and carrying out processes (Bich, 2018; Kirchhoff, Parr, Palacios, Friston, & Kiverstein, 2018). In this metabolic exchange, the RNA world acquired sufficient robustness in its physicochemical processes with which to adapt and maintain viability (Larhlimi, Blachon, Selbig, & Nikoloski, 2011). Equally, another fundamental factor was the origin of the symbiosis between RNA and proteins (where RNA synthesizes proteins and proteins synthesize RNA); in this molecular mutualism innovation, coevolution, resilience, and fitness were enhanced (Lanier, Petrov, & Williams, 2017). Likewise, in this acquisition of complexity in chemical signals, coevolution was achieved to the extent that the structures interact and it was in the molecular mutualism with the RNA that the mutation factor could include greater chemical and adaptive diversity in the process (López-García, Eme, & Moreira, 2017; Urano, Dong, Bennetzen, & Jones, 2015). Thus, proteins gave shape to the RNA world through communication and catalysis that allowed it to organize the initial biochemistry that established the foundation of biological functions (Harms & Thornton, 2013; van der Gulik & Speijer, 2015). In the same way, this coevolution has been demonstrated in the origin of the ribosomal RNA that arose from the given mutualism between RNA and proteins (Harish & Caetano-Anollés, 2012).

On the other hand, the passage of abiotic RNA to genetic RNA required interaction and communication; in this case, the cAMP from the ATP is considered an ancestral metabolic regulator, whose primordial function in chemical signaling allowed obtaining energy from the available sources (Banfalvi, 2019; Lehman, 2015). Likewise, cAMP is linked to the connection that unites the RNA world with the viral world in the emergence of the common cell ancestor, or LUCA (Jheeta, 2015); the ancestor that would also count on this messenger as a regulatory mechanism of gene expression, which provided a fundamental tool in the interaction with the environment (Dorman, Bhriain, & Dorman, 2018). Interactions of viruses and protocells that accumulated innovations led to the appearance of the first eukaryotic organisms (Fig. 2) (Koonin, 2016), due to the introduction of the viral mutation within the adaptation process that introduced changes in RNA, which led to a chemical diversity of metabolic pathways,

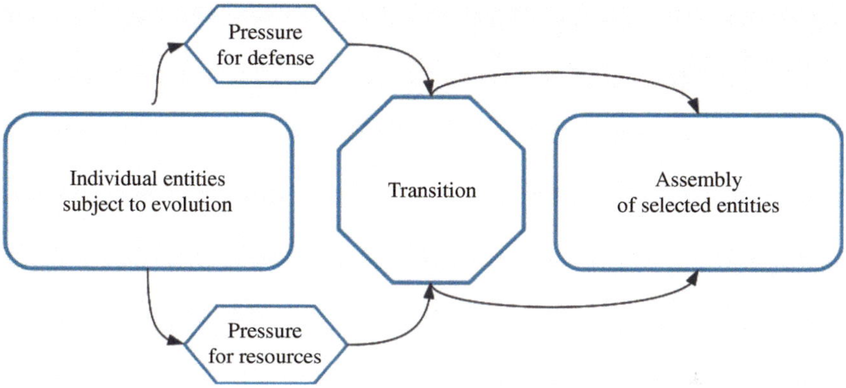

Fig. 2 Evolutionary transitions.

and this characteristic of genetic diversity to acquire fitness in survival persists in RNA viruses (Domingo, Sheldon, & Perales, 2012; Durzyńska & Goździcka-Józefiak, 2015).

Thus, this chemical coevolution of the interaction led to the configuration of more sophisticated communication networks such as the quorum sensing that allowed the establishment of communities of biological units that shared biological functions (Diggle, Gardner, West, & Griffin, 2007; Schluter, Schoech, Foster, & Mitri, 2016).

4.3 Chemical evolution and proteins: The first model

In this way, the interaction carried out by general-purpose multifunctional enzymes with the ability to catalyze several chemical reactions is another of the main factors within the chemical mutualism that allowed the synthesis of self-replicating molecules and with the ability to respond to environmental stimuli (Cheng et al., 2012; Newton, Arcus, Gerth, & Patrick, 2018). This coevolution between proteins and RNA, where the RNA template folded proteins from existing monomers to develop autocatalytic metabolic processes, was a key moment of mutualism and the transition from chemical to biological evolution (Czárán, Könnyű, & Szathmáry, 2015). In this way, in a world prior to the appearance of RNA, the processing of information and catalysis must have been carried out by protometabolic entities that subsequently were coupled to RNA. At this time, it is proposed that said entity is the ß-amyloid peptide (Maury, 2018). This amyloid peptide also has the ability to establish fibrillar networks capable of coupling and establishing interconnected structures of information sharing (Wei et al., 2017).

These fibrillar patterns grow through polymerization processes and are the basis of the polymorphism of these proteins (Tycko, 2014).

In this amyloid interactome, protein-protein interactions led to metabolic processes that acquired complexity of association and function that, upon entering into communication with the RNA world, achieved a self-sustaining state (Nevola & Giralt, 2015). Thus, due to the enzymatic promiscuity, evolutionary biochemistry gained robustness to maintain energy processes despite environmental challenges (Copley, 2015). Likewise, the metabolism not mediated by enzymes should be taken into account, in which metal cation, Fe (II), plays a fundamental role for obtaining energy, as evidenced in nonenzymatic glycolysis, which apparently was crucial for the appearance of metabolic pathways in conjunction with protein interactions and RNA (Ralser, 2018). In addition, the union of enzymatic promiscuity, as well as metabolism not mediated by enzymes, gave greater stability to the metabolic network allowing self-sustainability under stress conditions (Piedrafita, Keller, & Ralser, 2015), because both processes can modify the chemical reactivity and alter the metabolic flux for the protection of the protocells (Caetano-Anollés et al., 2009; Goldford & Segrè, 2018). So, these bases of protometabolism optimized the biochemical conditions for the genetic coding that later led to the appearance of LUCA and thus connect the prebiotic world with the biotic world (Kunnev & Gospodinov, 2018).

4.4 Multifunctional enzymes and the secondary metabolites explosion

Multifunctional enzymes capable of catalyzing chemical reactions with great promiscuity led to the consolidation of the protocell as a self-sustaining system and the development of a secondary metabolism (Hordijk, 2016; Hordijk & Steel, 2018). This facilitated the establishment of autocatalytic networks, exchange of information, and sharing of entropy through Darwinian optimization mechanisms, summarized as cooperation, fitness, and mutation (Fig. 3) (Schuster, 2016). These metabolic networks put in place the biogeochemistry of ecosystems in primitive microbial systems, where multifunctional enzymes would be key in the production of chemically diverse compounds for adaptation to different environments (Perez-Garcia, Lear, & Singhal, 2016; Vallino, 2010). In this way, multifunctional enzymes with a high degree of promiscuity for the processing of secondary metabolites were a driver of chemical diversity of molecules with biological activity, such as cytochrome P450, involved in the metabolism of terpenoid

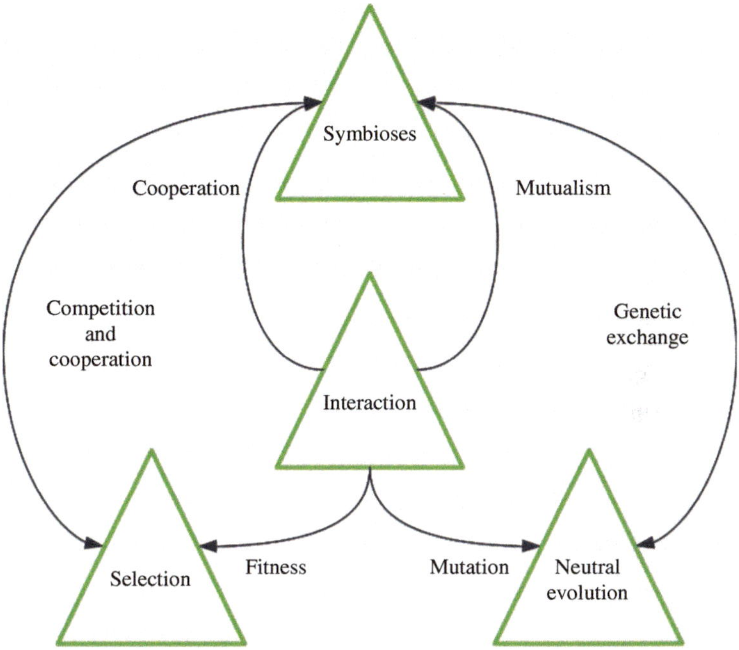

Fig. 3 Mechanisms of Darwinian optimization.

compounds (Bathe & Tissier, 2019). In addition, as a result of the interactions, the metabolites were specialized to carry out diverse biological functions in the metabolic pathways and this produced changes in the genetic information of LUCA as duplication and divergences of DNA sequences that drove the evolution of genes and genomes (Emiliani, Fondi, Liò, & Fani, 2010). Thus, in this search for homeostasis, all organisms established a network of proteostasis or equilibrium of enzymatic processes to facilitate the coevolution and adaptation of the proteome in the synthesis of specialized molecules, which also modulates both the structure of proteins and their function (Díaz-Villanueva, Díaz-Molina, & García-González, 2015; Powers & Balch, 2013). Equally, protein homeostasis regulates the synthesis of new peptides against environmental changes, allowing proteome adaptation (Arnsburg & Kirstein-Miles, 2014). Likewise, these genetic duplications and divergences allowed the consolidation of the bases of chemical diversity so far expressed in the superfamily of cytochromes P450 that control the routes of specialized metabolites in plants (Hamberger & Bak, 2013).

On the other hand, proteostasis is linked to DNA repair, so there is a connection between protein stability and mutagenesis, which is a chemical diversity driver that increases fitness (Xie & Jarosz, 2018). In this way, molecular chaperones such as Hsp90 can alleviate the effect of mutations and maintain balance in protein synthesis (Geller, Pechmann, Acevedo, Andino, & Frydman, 2018). In addition, Hsp90 is induced by environmental stress, increasing the production of secondary metabolites for survival, as observed in bacteria (Garcie et al., 2016). Furthermore, Hsp90 is susceptible to be inhibited by other metabolites so this could be an interesting therapeutic target for the development of new drugs (Dal Piaz, Terracciano, De Tommasi, & Braca, 2015).

Finally, the promiscuity of the multifunctional proteins influenced the biosynthetic gene clusters (BGCs) and their expression mechanisms, linking these genes to the modulation by their metabolites and synthesis pathways (Trautman & Crawford, 2016), configuring a global metabolic network that favors recombination, the explosion of diversity, cognition, and the ability to predict the environment (Reen, Romano, Dobson, & O'Gara, 2015; Wisecaver et al., 2017).

4.5 Cytochromes as enhancers of specialized metabolites

In the search for energy self-sustainability, a fundamental step was the use of oxygen for the aerobic generation of energy; in this aspect, bacterial cytochrome *c* oxidase (COX) has been crucial in the chemical evolution (Wikström, Krab, & Sharma, 2018). Thus, the metabolic activity of cytochrome *c* oxidase induces regulation by the secondary metabolism in order to optimize the use of energy, as observed in the Pasteur effect of fermentation (Barberel & Walker, 2000). This is how these mechanisms of metabolism modulation allow microorganisms to cope with environmental changes, through the production of antioxidant molecules and molecular communicators that exchange information with other microbial populations (Baez & Shiloach, 2014; Ruiz et al., 2010). Thus, the optimization of the use of carbon and oxygen sources has molded microbial metabolic responses to enter homeostasis inside the holobiont (Phelan, Liu, Pogliano, & Dorrestein, 2012). Likewise, reactive oxygen species and the oxidation-reduction balance can modulate the expression of BGCs in response to metabolic regulation in bacteria (Arakawa, 2018; Wang, Gao, & Tang, 2012). So in the evolution of cytochromes as transporters of chemical energy, the appearance of the cytochrome P450s (CYPs) family in the first prokaryotic cells opens the possibility of the synthesis of secondary metabolites that are more chemically diverse and with greater biological functions, such as terpenes and alkaloids (Greule, Stok, De Voss, & Cryle, 2018; Zhang et al., 2018). Likewise, cytochrome P450 enzymes expression can be epigenetically modulated through its catalyzed products, as well as the genes responsible for the biosynthesis of specialized metabolites, thereby increasing the capacity for response and adaptation to the environment (Tamási & Falus, 2012; Tang & Chen, 2015). Similarly, bacterial CYPs can associate with other enzymes with redox properties such as ferredoxin to produce secondary metabolites such as antibiotics and pigments (Child et al., 2018).

On the other hand, there is currently an increasing tendency to design microbial factories for the synthesis of secondary metabolites to obtain useful products; in this way, it has been demonstrated that not only BGCs are important for production, but also the different cytochromes are required to recreate biosynthetic pathways and thus synthesize molecules with biological activity, because they are the most diverse catalytic enzymes and an association has been identified between the greater presence of these enzymes and the expression of the BGCs (Li, Li, & Smolke, 2018; Mthethwa et al., 2018). This will be a field of intense research to unite genomics and metabolomics in which the design of metabolic models based on the insertion of synthetic genes can be an impact tool in the pharmaceutical industry (Nielsen & Nielsen, 2017).

4.6 The interaction between the environment and multifunctional enzymes: Adaptation in chemical diversity

The evolution of biosynthetic pathways depends on a constant balance between environmental changes and the adaptations that the complex biological system makes, whose response is evoked by the multifunctional enzymes that it has (Trastoy et al., 2018). Likewise, the coevolution of biosynthesis allows the production of molecules with biological activity to establish communication and exchange networks that interact with highly promiscuous enzymes (Livnat, 2013). Thus, in this dynamic evolution, enzymes acquire adaptive capacity as they catalyze a greater number of chemical reactions and transform different substrates with the same catalytic process (Cuesta, Rahman, Furnham, & Thornton, 2015; Kaltenbach & Tokuriki, 2014). However, acquiring fitness to develop optimal enzymatic reactions that are beneficial to the biological system is as important as adapting (Wohlgemuth, 2018). In this game of gain and loss of function, it becomes a priority to maintain the thermodynamic equilibrium of the metabolic network in order to move from preadaptations, or exaptations, to innovation and evolution (Sambamoorthy, Sinha, & Raman, 2019), assuming innovation as the ability to develop new metabolic pathways using combinations of enzymes originated through horizontal gene transfer, change in the regulation of existing enzymes, as well as modifications in the amino acid sequences that originate new enzymatic functions (Prosser, Larrouy-Maumus, & de Carvalho, 2014; Wagner, 2011). Thus, in this process of enzymatic recruitment resulting from random mutations, new beneficial functions can be acquired for the host organism, and that promotes the expansion of metabolic activities (Schulenburg & Miller, 2014).

On the other hand, the phenomenon of enzymatic recruitment can modify the chemical signaling between the communities belonging to the biological system, thus promoting new metabolic pathways that allow persistence (Davies & Davies, 2010; Moradali, Ghods, & Rehm, 2017). The ability to experimentally induce the evolution and innovation of metabolic pathways to obtain new chemically diverse metabolites is one of the possibilities of interaction and communication for adaptation (Nam, Conrad, & Lewis, 2011; Pandit, Srinivasan, & Mahadevan, 2017). Thus, the study of metabolic interactions in response to environmental changes will have the ability to avoid reductionism as well as to know the functioning of biological systems in order to discover new applications and develop innovations (Roukos, 2011).

4.7 Symbiosis: The role of the holobiont as a source of chemical evolution

Thus the symbiosis as a driver of the evolution of metabolic pathways allows the molecular exchange of metabolites through chemical signals that share the information and determine the biological activity of the synthesized compounds (Medlock et al., 2018; Ponomarova et al., 2017). Likewise, the genetic exchange within the holobiont allows the evolution of enzymes and increases their promiscuity; that is, it promotes the acquisition of functions (Copley, 2017; Seelig, 2017), achieving with this the hologenomic change that drives the efficiency of the production of metabolites by specialized enzymatic processes (O'Brien, Webster, Miller, & Bourne, 2019). In addition, the communication between the host and the microbiota and their mutualist symbiosis optimizes the use of energy sources, as well as obtaining the essential nutrients for the synthesis of the molecules of life (McFall-Ngai et al., 2013; Ohland & Jobin, 2015). The evolution of the enzymes is fundamental to maintain the homeostasis of the holobiont and, in this way, the dysbiosis through the modification of the chemical signals interrupts the functionality in metabolic processes driving the enzymatic networks to catalyze harmful reactions for the biological system (Dicks, Geldenhuys, Mikkelsen, Brandsborg, & Marcotte, 2018; Putignani & Dallapiccola, 2016). On the other hand, the adaptations of the metabolic networks in the disease processes can be successful and develop new synthetic pathways that induce the persistence of the holobiont; this is possible thanks to the robustness acquired in the redundancy of the genes that express the enzymes that regulate these processes (Edwards, 2017; He, Fromion, & Westerhoff, 2013). In this way, the chemical evolution has been shaped from the interactions between biological systems and unites diversity with communication and fitness in the way of survival (Vane-Wright, 2018).

4.8 Conclusions

The evolution of the biosynthesis of new and varied metabolites is a union between adaptation and innovation, and forms the basis of the chemical diversity present in the biosphere (Dias, Urban, & Roessner, 2012; Malve, 2016). Thus, chemical evolution has increased in complexity from the transition of the abiotic world to become a fundamental tool of the biotic world, both in response to environmental changes and to induce mutation (Voje, Holen, Liow, & Stenseth, 2015). In this way, the complexity of the biotic world was acquired through the capacity to catalyze as many substrates as possible and to establish sufficient metabolic networks to favor the host (Egel, 2012). Thus the chemical evolution opens the possibility of inducing experimental evolution in order to obtain new chemically diverse products (D'Souza & Kost, 2016). Likewise, chemical evolution through enzymatic promiscuity can be used as an innovation model for the production of new biotechnological products from bacteria and fungi (Arnold, 2015, 2018a, 2018b). Finally, it is necessary to study biosynthesis networks in their entire complexity by integrating into a meta-omic model the different manifestations of interactions in action (Zuñiga, Zaramela, & Zengler, 2017).

References

Abusnina, A., & Lugnier, C. (2017). Therapeutic potentials of natural compounds acting on cyclic nucleotide phosphodiesterase families. *Cellular Signalling*, *39*, 55–65.

Arakawa, K. (2018). Manipulation of metabolic pathways controlled by signaling molecules, inducers of antibiotic production, for genome mining in *Streptomyces* spp. *Antonie van Leeuwenhoek*, *111*(5), 743–751.

Arnold, F. H. (2015). The nature of chemical innovation: New enzymes by evolution. *Quarterly Reviews of Biophysics*, *48*(4), 404–410.

Arnold, F. H. (2018a). Directed evolution: Bringing new chemistry to life. *Angewandte Chemie International Edition*, *57*(16), 4143–4148.

Arnold, F. H. (2018b). Enzymes by evolution: Bringing new chemistry to life. *Molecular Frontiers Journal*, *2*(01), 9–18.

Arnsburg, K., & Kirstein-Miles, J. (2014). Interrelation between protein synthesis, proteostasis and life span. *Current Genomics*, *15*(1), 66–75.

Baez, A., & Shiloach, J. (2014). Effect of elevated oxygen concentration on bacteria, yeasts, and cells propagated for production of biological compounds. *Microbial Cell Factories*, *13*(1), 181.

Banfalvi, G. (2019). Origin of coding RNA from random-sequence RNA. *DNA and Cell Biology*, *38*(3), 223–228.

Barberel, S. I., & Walker, J. R. (2000). The effect of aeration upon the secondary metabolism of microorganisms. *Biotechnology and Genetic Engineering Reviews*, *17*(1), 281–326.

Bathe, U., & Tissier, A. (2019). Cytochrome P450 enzymes: A driving force of plant diterpene diversity. *Phytochemistry*.

Beran, F., Köllner, T. G., Gershenzon, J., & Tholl, D. (2019). Chemical convergence between plants and insects: Biosynthetic origins and functions of common secondary metabolites. *New Phytologist*.

Bich, L. (2018). Robustness and autonomy in biological systems: How regulatory mechanisms enable functional integration, complexity and minimal cognition through the action of second-order control constraints. In M. Bertolaso, S. Caianiello, & E. Serrelli (Eds.), *Biological robustness* (pp. 123–147). Cham: Springer.

Brodie, J., Ball, S. G., Bouget, F. Y., Chan, C. X., De Clerck, O., Cock, J. M., … Saha, M. (2017). Biotic interactions as drivers of algal origin and evolution. *New Phytologist*, *216*(3), 670–681.

Caetano-Anollés, G., Yafremava, L. S., Gee, H., Caetano-Anollés, D., Kim, H. S., & Mittenthal, J. E. (2009). The origin and evolution of modern metabolism. *The International Journal of Biochemistry & Cell Biology*, *41*(2), 285–297.

Chen, X., Köllner, T. G., Jia, Q., Norris, A., Santhanam, B., Rabe, P., … Chen, F. (2016). Terpene synthase genes in eukaryotes beyond plants and fungi: Occurrence in social amoebae. *Proceedings of the National Academy of Sciences*, *113*(43), 12132–12137.

Cheng, X. Y., Huang, W. J., Hu, S. C., Zhang, H. L., Wang, H., Zhang, J. X., … Ji, Z. L. (2012). A global characterization and identification of multifunctional enzymes. *PLoS ONE*, *7*(6), e38979.

Chezem, W. R., & Clay, N. K. (2016). Regulation of plant secondary metabolism and associated specialized cell development by MYBs and bHLHs. *Phytochemistry*, *131*, 26–43.

Child, S. A., Bradley, J. M., Pukala, T. L., Svistunenko, D. A., Le Brun, N. E., & Bell, S. G. (2018). Electron transfer ferredoxins with unusual cluster binding motifs support secondary metabolism in many bacteria. *Chemical Science*, *9*(41), 7948–7957.

Copley, S. D. (2015). An evolutionary biochemist's perspective on promiscuity. *Trends in Biochemical Sciences*, *40*(2), 72–78.

Copley, S. D. (2017). Shining a light on enzyme promiscuity. *Current Opinion in Structural Biology*, *47*, 167–175.

Cuesta, S. M., Rahman, S. A., Furnham, N., & Thornton, J. M. (2015). The classification and evolution of enzyme function. *Biophysical Journal*, *109*(6), 1082–1086.

Czárán, T., Könnyű, B., & Szathmáry, E. (2015). Metabolically coupled replicator systems: Overview of an RNA-world model concept of prebiotic evolution on mineral surfaces. *Journal of Theoretical Biology*, *381*, 39–54.

D'Souza, G., & Kost, C. (2016). Experimental evolution of metabolic dependency in bacteria. *PLoS Genetics*, *12*(11), e1006364.

Dal Piaz, F., Terracciano, S., De Tommasi, N., & Braca, A. (2015). Hsp90 activity modulation by plant secondary metabolites. *Planta Medica*, *81*(14), 1223–1239.

Davies, J., & Davies, D. (2010). Origins and evolution of antibiotic resistance. *Microbiology and Molecular Biology Reviews*, 74(3), 417–433.

Dias, D. A., Urban, S., & Roessner, U. (2012). A historical overview of natural products in drug discovery. *Metabolites*, *2*(2), 303–336.

Díaz-Villanueva, J., Díaz-Molina, R., & García-González, V. (2015). Protein folding and mechanisms of proteostasis. *International Journal of Molecular Sciences*, *16*(8), 17193–17230.

Dicks, L. M. T., Geldenhuys, J., Mikkelsen, L. S., Brandsborg, E., & Marcotte, H. (2018). Our gut microbiota: A long walk to homeostasis. *Beneficial Microbes*, *9*(1), 3–20.

Diggle, S. P., Gardner, A., West, S. A., & Griffin, A. S. (2007). Evolutionary theory of bacterial quorum sensing: When is a signal not a signal? *Philosophical Transactions of the Royal Society, B: Biological Sciences*, *362*(1483), 1241–1249.

Domingo, E., Sheldon, J., & Perales, C. (2012). Viral quasispecies evolution. *Microbiology and Molecular Biology Reviews*, *76*(2), 159–216.

Dorman, C. J., Bhriain, N. N., & Dorman, M. J. (2018). The evolution of gene regulatory mechanisms in bacteria. In P. H. Rampelotto (Ed.), *Molecular mechanisms of microbial evolution* (pp. 125–152). Cham: Springer.

Durzyńska, J., & Goździcka-Józefiak, A. (2015). Viruses and cells intertwined since the dawn of evolution. *Virology Journal*, *12*(1), 169.

Edwards, L. M. (2017). Metabolic systems biology: A brief primer. *The Journal of Physiology*, *595*(9), 2849–2855.

Egel, R. (2012). Life's order, complexity, organization, and its thermodynamic–holistic imperatives. *Life*, *2*(4), 323–363.

Emiliani, G., Fondi, M., Liò, P., & Fani, R. (2010). Evolution of metabolic pathways and evolution of genomes. In A. Loi, M. Mandl, & L. L. Barton (Eds.), *Geomicrobiology: Molecular and environmental perspective* (pp. 37–68). Dordrecht: Springer.

Garcie, C., Tronnet, S., Garénaux, A., McCarthy, A. J., Brachmann, A. O., Pénary, M., … Dozois, C. M. (2016). The bacterial stress-responsive Hsp90 chaperone (HtpG) is required for the production of the genotoxin colibactin and the siderophore yersiniabactin in *Escherichia coli*. *The Journal of Infectious Diseases*, *214*(6), 916–924.

Geller, R., Pechmann, S., Acevedo, A., Andino, R., & Frydman, J. (2018). Hsp90 shapes protein and RNA evolution to balance trade-offs between protein stability and aggregation. *Nature Communications*, *9*(1), 1781.

Goldford, J. E., & Segrè, D. (2018). Modern views of ancient metabolic networks. *Current Opinion in Systems Biology*, *8*, 117–124.

Greule, A., Stok, J. E., De Voss, J. J., & Cryle, M. J. (2018). Unrivalled diversity: The many roles and reactions of bacterial cytochromes P450 in secondary metabolism. *Natural Product Reports*, *35*(8), 757–791.

Hamberger, B., & Bak, S. (2013). Plant P450s as versatile drivers for evolution of species-specific chemical diversity. *Philosophical Transactions of the Royal Society, B: Biological Sciences*, *368*(1612), 20120426.

Harish, A., & Caetano-Anollés, G. (2012). Ribosomal history reveals origins of modern protein synthesis. *PLoS ONE*, 7(3), e32776.

Harms, M. J., & Thornton, J. W. (2013). Evolutionary biochemistry: Revealing the historical and physical causes of protein properties. *Nature Reviews Genetics*, *14*(8), 559.

Hauryliuk, V., Atkinson, G. C., Murakami, K. S., Tenson, T., & Gerdes, K. (2015). Recent functional insights into the role of (p) ppGpp in bacterial physiology. *Nature Reviews Microbiology*, *13*(5), 298.

He, F., Fromion, V., & Westerhoff, H. V. (2013). (Im) perfect robustness and adaptation of metabolic networks subject to metabolic and gene-expression regulation: Marrying control engineering with metabolic control analysis. *BMC Systems Biology*, 7(1), 131.

Hengge, R., Häussler, S., Pruteanu, M., Stülke, J., Tschowri, N., & Turgay, K. (2019). Recent advances and current trends in nucleotide second messenger signaling in bacteria. *Journal of Molecular Biology*, *431*, 908–927.
Hernández-Morales, R., Becerra, A., & Lazcano, A. (2019). Alarmones as vestiges of a bygone RNA world. *Journal of Molecular Evolution*, *87*(1), 37–51.
Higgs, P. G., & Lehman, N. (2015). The RNA world: Molecular cooperation at the origins of life. *Nature Reviews Genetics*, *16*(1), 7.
Hordijk, W. (2016). Evolution of autocatalytic sets in computational models of chemical reaction networks. *Origins of Life and Evolution of Biospheres*, *46*(2–3), 233–245.
Hordijk, W., & Steel, M. (2018). Autocatalytic networks at the basis of life's origin and organization. *Life*, *8*(4), 62.
Hud, N.V. (2018). Searching for lost nucleotides of the pre-RNA world with a self-refining model of early Earth. *Nature Communications*, *9*, .
Jheeta, S. (2015). The routes of emergence of life from LUCA during the RNA and viral world: A conspectus. *Life*, *5*(2), 1445–1453.
Kaltenbach, M., & Tokuriki, N. (2014). Dynamics and constraints of enzyme evolution. *Journal of Experimental Zoology Part B: Molecular and Developmental Evolution*, *322*(7), 468–487.
Kirchhoff, M., Parr, T., Palacios, E., Friston, K., & Kiverstein, J. (2018). The Markov blankets of life: Autonomy, active inference and the free energy principle. *Journal of the Royal Society Interface*, *15*(138), 20170792.
Kitadai, N., & Maruyama, S. (2018). Origins of building blocks of life: A review. *Geoscience Frontiers*, *9*(4), 1117–1153.
Koonin, E. V. (2016). Viruses and mobile elements as drivers of evolutionary transitions. *Philosophical Transactions of the Royal Society, B: Biological Sciences*, *371*(1701), 20150442.
Kunnev, D., & Gospodinov, A. (2018). Possible emergence of sequence specific RNA aminoacylation via peptide intermediary to initiate Darwinian evolution and code through origin of life. *Life*, *8*(4), 44.
Lange, B. M. (2015). The evolution of plant secretory structures and emergence of terpenoid chemical diversity. *Annual Review of Plant Biology*, *66*, 139–159.
Lanier, K. A., Petrov, A. S., & Williams, L. D. (2017). The central symbiosis of molecular biology: Molecules in mutualism. *Journal of Molecular Evolution*, *85*(1–2), 8–13.
Larhlimi, A., Blachon, S., Selbig, J., & Nikoloski, Z. (2011). Robustness of metabolic networks: A review of existing definitions. *Biosystems*, *106*(1), 1–8.
Lawrence, D., Fiegna, F., Behrends, V., Bundy, J. G., Phillimore, A. B., Bell, T., & Barraclough, T. G. (2012). Species interactions alter evolutionary responses to a novel environment. *PLoS Biology*, *10*(5), e1001330.
Lehman, N. (2015). The RNA world: 4,000,000,050 years old. *Life*, *5*(4), 1583.
Li, S., Li, Y., & Smolke, C. D. (2018). Strategies for microbial synthesis of high-value phytochemicals. *Nature Chemistry*, *10*(4), 395–404.
Livnat, A. (2013). Interaction-based evolution: How natural selection and nonrandom mutation work together. *Biology Direct*, *8*(1), 24.
López-García, P., Eme, L., & Moreira, D. (2017). Symbiosis in eukaryotic evolution. *Journal of Theoretical Biology*, *434*, 20–33.
Malve, H. (2016). Exploring the ocean for new drug developments: Marine pharmacology. *Journal of Pharmacy & Bioallied Sciences*, *8*(2), 83.
Maury, C. P. J. (2018). Amyloid and the origin of life: Self-replicating catalytic amyloids as prebiotic informational and protometabolic entities. *Cellular and Molecular Life Sciences*, *75*(9), 1499–1507.
McFall-Ngai, M., Hadfield, M. G., Bosch, T. C., Carey, H. V., Domazet-Lošo, T., Douglas, A. E., … Hentschel, U. (2013). Animals in a bacterial world, a new imperative for the life sciences. *Proceedings of the National Academy of Sciences*, *110*(9), 3229–3236.

Medlock, G. L., Carey, M. A., McDuffie, D. G., Mundy, M. B., Giallourou, N., Swann, J. R., … Papin, J. A. (2018). Inferring metabolic mechanisms of interaction within a defined gut microbiota. *Cell Systems*, *7*(3), 245–257.

Moradali, M. F., Ghods, S., & Rehm, B. H. (2017). *Pseudomonas aeruginosa* lifestyle: A paradigm for adaptation, survival, and persistence. *Frontiers in Cellular and Infection Microbiology*, *7*, 39.

Mthethwa, B., Chen, W., Ngwenya, M., Kappo, A., Syed, P., Karpoormath, R., … Syed, K. (2018). Comparative analyses of cytochrome P450s and those associated with secondary metabolism in *Bacillus* species. *International Journal of Molecular Sciences*, *19*(11), 3623.

Nam, H., Conrad, T., & Lewis, N. E. (2011). Metabolic pathway evolution and cellular objectives. *Current Opinion in Biotechnology*, *22*(4), 595.

Nelson, J. W., & Breaker, R. R. (2017). The lost language of the RNA world. *Sci Signal*, *10*(483), eaam8812.

Nevola, L., & Giralt, E. (2015). Modulating protein–protein interactions: The potential of peptides. *Chemical Communications*, *51*(16), 3302–3315.

Newton, M. S., Arcus, V. L., Gerth, M. L., & Patrick, W. M. (2018). Enzyme evolution: Innovation is easy, optimization is complicated. *Current Opinion in Structural Biology*, *48*, 110–116.

Nielsen, J. C., & Nielsen, J. (2017). Development of fungal cell factories for the production of secondary metabolites: Linking genomics and metabolism. *Synthetic and Systems Biotechnology*, *2*(1), 5–12.

O'Brien, P. A., Webster, N. S., Miller, D. J., & Bourne, D. G. (2019). Host-microbe coevolution: Applying evidence from model systems to complex marine invertebrate holobionts. *mBio*, *10*(1), e02241-18.

O'Flaherty, D. K., Kamat, N. P., Mirza, F. N., Li, L., Prywes, N., & Szostak, J. W. (2018). Copying of mixed-sequence RNA templates inside model protocells. *Journal of the American Chemical Society*, *140*(15), 5171–5178.

Ohland, C. L., & Jobin, C. (2015). Microbial activities and intestinal homeostasis: A delicate balance between health and disease. *Cellular and Molecular Gastroenterology and Hepatology*, *1*(1), 28–40.

Pandit, A. V., Srinivasan, S., & Mahadevan, R. (2017). Redesigning metabolism based on orthogonality principles. *Nature Communications*, *8*, 15188.

Pechuan, X., Puzio, R., & Bergman, A. (2018). The evolutionary dynamics of metabolic protocells. *PLoS Computational Biology*, *14*(7), e1006265.

Perez-Garcia, O., Lear, G., & Singhal, N. (2016). Metabolic network modeling of microbial interactions in natural and engineered environmental systems. *Frontiers in Microbiology*, *7*, 673.

Phelan, V. V., Liu, W. T., Pogliano, K., & Dorrestein, P. C. (2012). Microbial metabolic exchange—The chemotype-to-phenotype link. *Nature Chemical Biology*, *8*(1), 26.

Pichersky, E., & Raguso, R. A. (2018). Why do plants produce so many terpenoid compounds? *New Phytologist*, *220*(3), 692–702.

Piedrafita, G., Keller, M., & Ralser, M. (2015). The impact of non-enzymatic reactions and enzyme promiscuity on cellular metabolism during (oxidative) stress conditions. *Biomolecules*, *5*(3), 2101–2122.

Ponomarova, O., Gabrielli, N., Sévin, D. C., Mülleder, M., Zirngibl, K., Bulyha, K., … Ralser, M. (2017). Yeast creates a niche for symbiotic lactic acid bacteria through nitrogen overflow. *Cell Systems*, *5*(4), 345–357.

Powers, E. T., & Balch, W. E. (2013). Diversity in the origins of proteostasis networks—A driver for protein function in evolution. *Nature Reviews Molecular Cell Biology*, *14*(4), 237.

Pross, A., & Pascal, R. (2017). How and why kinetics, thermodynamics, and chemistry induce the logic of biological evolution. *Beilstein Journal of Organic Chemistry*, *13*(1), 665–674.

Prosser, G. A., Larrouy-Maumus, G., & de Carvalho, L. P. S. (2014). Metabolomic strategies for the identification of new enzyme functions and metabolic pathways. *EMBO Reports*, *15*(6), 657–669.

Putignani, L., & Dallapiccola, B. (2016). Foodomics as part of the host-microbiota-exposome interplay. *Journal of Proteomics*, *147*, 3–20.

Ralser, M. (2018). An appeal to magic? The discovery of a non-enzymatic metabolism and its role in the origins of life. *Biochemical Journal*, *475*(16), 2577–2592.

Reen, F., Romano, S., Dobson, A., & O'Gara, F. (2015). The sound of silence: Activating silent biosynthetic gene clusters in marine microorganisms. *Marine Drugs*, *13*(8), 4754–4783.

Roukos, D. H. (2011). Networks medicine: From reductionism to evidence of complex dynamic biomolecular interactions. *Pharmacogenomics*, *12*(5), 695–698.

Ruiz, B., Chávez, A., Forero, A., García-Huante, Y., Romero, A., Sánchez, M., … Langley, E. (2010). Production of microbial secondary metabolites: Regulation by the carbon source. *Critical Reviews in Microbiology*, *36*(2), 146–167.

Ruiz-Mirazo, K., Briones, C., & de la Escosura, A. (2017). Chemical roots of biological evolution: The origins of life as a process of development of autonomous functional systems. *Open Biology*, 7(4), 170050.

Sambamoorthy, G., Sinha, H., & Raman, K. (2019). Evolutionary design principles in metabolism. *Proceedings of the Royal Society B*, *286*(1898), 20190098.

Schluter, J., Schoech, A. P., Foster, K. R., & Mitri, S. (2016). The evolution of quorum sensing as a mechanism to infer kinship. *PLoS Computational Biology*, *12*(4), e1004848.

Schulenburg, C., & Miller, B. G. (2014). Enzyme recruitment and its role in metabolic expansion. *Biochemistry*, *53*(5), 836–845.

Schuster, P. (2016). Increase in complexity and information through molecular evolution. *Entropy*, *18*(11), 397.

Seelig, B. (2017). Multifunctional enzymes from reduced genomes–model proteins for simple primordial metabolism? *Molecular Microbiology*, *105*(4), 505–507.

Solé, R. (2016). Synthetic transitions: Towards a new synthesis. *Philosophical Transactions of the Royal Society, B: Biological Sciences*, *371*(1701), 20150438.

Szappanos, B., Fritzemeier, J., Csörgő, B., Lázár, V., Lu, X., Fekete, G., … Lercher, M. J. (2016). Adaptive evolution of complex innovations through stepwise metabolic niche expansion. *Nature Communications*, 7, 11607.

Tamási, V., & Falus, A. (2012). Genetic and epigenetic factors affecting cytochrome P450 phenotype and their clinical relevance. In J. Paxton (Ed.), *Topics on drug metabolism* (pp. 87–110). London: IntechOpen.

Tang, X., & Chen, S. (2015). Epigenetic regulation of cytochrome P450 enzymes and clinical implication. *Current Drug Metabolism*, *16*(2), 86–96.

Trastoy, R., Manso, T., Fernandez-Garcia, L., Blasco, L., Ambroa, A., Del Molino, M. P., … Tomas, M. (2018). Mechanisms of bacterial tolerance and persistence in the gastrointestinal and respiratory environments. *Clinical Microbiology Reviews*, *31*(4), e00023-18.

Trautman, E. P., & Crawford, J. M. (2016). Linking biosynthetic gene clusters to their metabolites via pathway-targeted molecular networking. *Current Topics in Medicinal Chemistry*, *16*(15), 1705–1716.

Tycko, R. (2014). Physical and structural basis for polymorphism in amyloid fibrils. *Protein Science*, *23*(11), 1528–1539.

Urano, D., Dong, T., Bennetzen, J. L., & Jones, A. M. (2015). Adaptive evolution of signaling partners. *Molecular Biology and Evolution*, *32*(4), 998–1007.

Vallino, J. J. (2010). Ecosystem biogeochemistry considered as a distributed metabolic network ordered by maximum entropy production. *Philosophical Transactions of the Royal Society, B: Biological Sciences*, *365*(1545), 1417–1427.

van der Gulik, P., & Speijer, D. (2015). How amino acids and peptides shaped the RNA world. *Life*, *5*(1), 230–246.

Vane-Wright, R. I. (2018). Agency, meaning, perception and mimicry: Perspectives from the process of life and third way of evolution. *Biosemiotics*, 1–21.

Villarreal, L. P., & Witzany, G. (2019). That is life: Communicating RNA networks from viruses and cells in continuous interaction. *Annals of the New York Academy of Sciences*, *40*, 1–16.

Voje, K. L., Holen, Ø.H., Liow, L. H., & Stenseth, N. C. (2015). The role of biotic forces in driving macroevolution: Beyond the Red Queen. *Proceedings of the Royal Society B: Biological Sciences*, *282*(1808), 20150186.

Wagner, A. (2011). The molecular origins of evolutionary innovations. *Trends in Genetics*, *27*(10), 397–410.

Wang, P., Gao, X., & Tang, Y. (2012). Complexity generation during natural product biosynthesis using redox enzymes. *Current Opinion in Chemical Biology*, *16*(3–4), 362–369.

Wang, J., Liu, K., Xing, R., & Yan, X. (2016). Peptide self-assembly: Thermodynamics and kinetics. *Chemical Society Reviews*, *45*(20), 5589–5604.

Wei, G., Su, Z., Reynolds, N. P., Arosio, P., Hamley, I. W., Gazit, E., & Mezzenga, R. (2017). Self-assembling peptide and protein amyloids: From structure to tailored function in nanotechnology. *Chemical Society Reviews*, *46*(15), 4661–4708.

Wikström, M., Krab, K., & Sharma, V. (2018). Oxygen activation and energy conservation by cytochrome c oxidase. *Chemical Reviews*, *118*(5), 2469–2490.

Wilke, C. O. (2012). Bringing molecules back into molecular evolution. *PLoS Computational Biology*, *8*(6), e1002572.

Wisecaver, J. H., Borowsky, A. T., Tzin, V., Jander, G., Kliebenstein, D. J., & Rokas, A. (2017). A global coexpression network approach for connecting genes to specialized metabolic pathways in plants. *The Plant Cell*, *29*(5), 944–959.

Wohlgemuth, R. (2018). Horizons of systems biocatalysis and renaissance of metabolite synthesis. *Biotechnology Journal*, *13*(6), 1700620.

Xie, J. L., & Jarosz, D. F. (2018). Mutations, protein homeostasis, and epigenetic control of genome integrity. *DNA Repair*, *71*, 23–32.

Zhang, W., Du, L., Li, F., Zhang, X., Qu, Z., Han, L., … Sun, Y. (2018). Mechanistic insights into interactions between bacterial class I P450 enzymes and redox partners. *ACS Catalysis*, *8*(11), 9992–10003.

Zuñiga, C., Zaramela, L., & Zengler, K. (2017). Elucidation of complexity and prediction of interactions in microbial communities. *Microbial Biotechnology*, *10*(6), 1500–1522.

CHAPTER 5
Autopoietic symbiogenesis in secondary metabolism

The mutual-aid tendency in man has so remote an origin, and is so deeply interwoven with all the past evolution of the human race, that is has been maintained by mankind up to the present time, notwithstanding all vicissitudes of history

In The Descent of Man he gave some powerful pages to illustrate its proper, wide sense. He pointed out how, in numberless animal societies, the struggle between separate individuals for the means of existence disappears, how struggle is replaced by co-operation, and how that substitution results in the development of intellectual and moral faculties which secure to the species the best conditions for survival.

in the long run the practice of solidarity proves much more advantageous to the species than the development of individuals endowed with predatory inclinations.

Piotr Kropotkin (1842–1921)

5.1 Introduction

The abundance and diversity of secondary metabolites is the result of the interactions present in the symbiotic networks that are established for the sharing of entropy in the complex biological system (Tianero et al., 2015). Likewise, the information for the expression of enzymes responsible for the production of metabolites is encoded in biosynthetic gene clusters, whose epigenetic regulation is mediated by environmental changes in order to allow adaptation and fitness in the stress phases (Fig. 1) (Etchegaray & Mostoslavsky, 2016; Steinberg, Stürzenbaum, & Menzel, 2008). Thus, the function of secondary metabolites in protecting against cell stress that favors interaction and symbiotic exchange has allowed the evolution of biological activities that allow establishing the communities of living beings

Molecular Evolutionary Models in Drug Discovery
https://doi.org/10.1016/B978-0-12-817613-9.00005-5

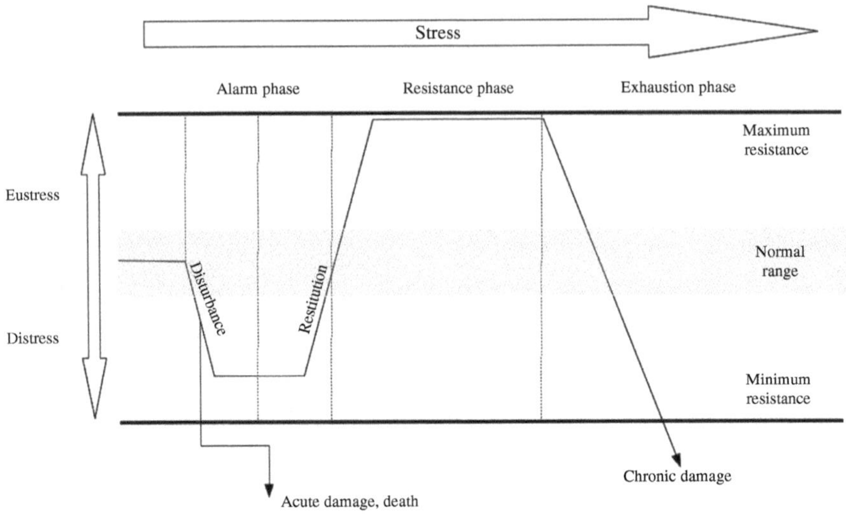

Fig. 1 Model of stress phases.

(Muraille, 2018; Rizzo & Lo Giudice, 2018). In addition, this symbiogenesis process of natural products (NPs) gives robustness and predictive capacity to the system, because it increases its ability to share chemical information through its molecular communicators (Boudouresque, Caumette, Bertrand, Normand, & Sime-Ngando, 2015; Lynch et al., 2014); for this reason, symbiosis originates in the same way: the symbiosis is autopoietic (Debernardi & Serrelli, 2013). This evolution of the symbiosis in its functionality has increased at the same time as the obtaining of products of the metabolism for the use of energy sources and adaptation to the ecosystem (Bueno, 2018; Guerrero & Berlanga, 2016).

In this way, the acquisition of fitness from the exchange of information mediated by the biological activity of secondary metabolites is only possible due to mutualism, which leads to the establishment of metabolic networks that benefit the species involved (Cavaliere, Feng, Soyer, & Jiménez, 2017; Leigh Jr., 2010). Likewise, the result of the sharing of chemical signals is the conformation of a holobiontic unit capable of evolving as its hologenome changes in response to changes in the ecosystem (Haag, 2018; Suárez, 2018). So the symbiopoiesis of the holobiont is the one that guarantees its self-replication and self-sustainability as a unit that establishes metabolic connections within a biological system that allows it to evolve in conjunction with its ecosystem (Gilbert, 2014; Sudakaran, Kost, & Kaltenpoth, 2017). Likewise, the secondary metabolism, by optimizing chemical communication in defense of space and the use of energy, achieved the functional symbiosis that in mutualism helped the establishment of metaorganisms (Schmidt, 2015; Schmidt, Donia, McIntosh, Fricke, & Ravel, 2012). So the objective of this chapter is to analyze the symbiosis as an autopoietic unit that uses secondary metabolism and its biological functions for the establishment of chemical signaling networks with which to configure a homeostatic equilibrium between the holobiont and the ecosystem; this is in order to design biotechnological applications that allow the development of innovations and apply the possibilities of the hologenome metabolomics (Bang et al., 2018).

5.2 Secondary metabolism in interactions and mutualism

The secondary metabolism, as well as the diversity of biological activities that it performs as a regulator, promoter, and optimizer of host interactions with the environment, has evolved in mutualism (Fig. 2) (Keller, 2018; Wichard & Beemelmanns, 2018). Mutualism in symbiotic interactions mediated by chemically diverse secondary metabolites allows metabolic networks of information exchange, association, and chemical evolution to be configured (Fukui, 2014; Wang & Seyedsayamdost, 2017). Thus, these signals activate biosynthetic pathways that regulate, modulate, and induce the production of bioactive molecules through the expression of the enzymes encoded in the BGCs, as well as cytochromes (Stringlis, Zhang, Pieterse, Bolton, & de Jonge, 2018; Wisecaver et al., 2017). Similarly, the secondary metabolites also

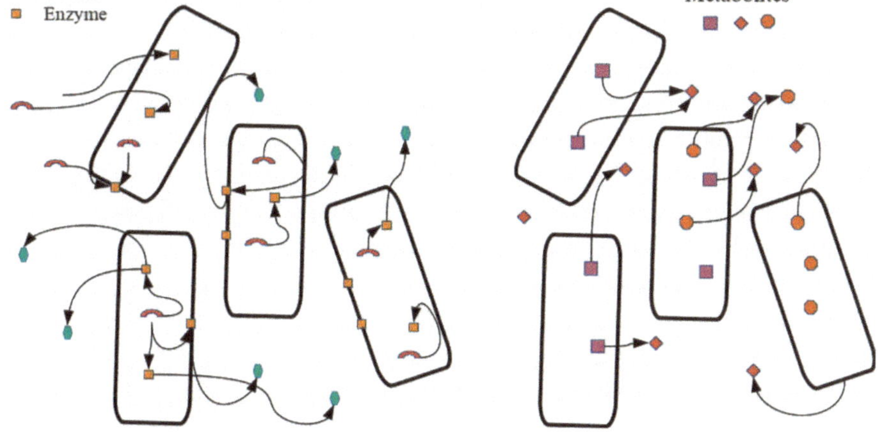

Fig. 2 Interaction and cooperation in secondary metabolism.

modulate the epigenetic control of the expression of the biosynthetic genes, activating or deactivating silent genes, as well as modulating the protein assembly (Leitão & Enguita, 2014; Quin, Flynn, & Schmidt-Dannert, 2014).

In this way, the secondary metabolism is an expression of the evolution of life in the biosphere by transferring information within the biological system in the framework of a mutualistic interaction (Kazamia, Helliwell, Purton, & Smith, 2016; Vitas & Dobovišek, 2018). So a living system is consolidated as a biological system when it establishes a secondary metabolism that regulates the obtaining of energy and exchanges chemical information with the ecosystem (Lucia, 2015; Terra & Passador, 2016). Additionally, chemical signaling mediated by bioactive compounds facilitates mutation and evolution by allowing exchange and genetic insertion in the hologenome (Kaessmann, 2010; Miller, 2016). So we are talking about the secondary metabolism as a source of cognition, self-reference, and self-replication of the biological system (Miller Jr., 2018; Razeto-Barry, 2012). In this way, if the secondary metabolites transfer chemical information and energy, they acquire the characteristic of modulating the biological systems to reach a homeostatic equilibrium that allows survival (Epstein, 2018; Vergara et al., 2019). Thus, molecular communicators as a biological information system modulate the adaptation, as well as the change and fitness, of the biological unit (Tu & Rappel, 2018). For this reason, the homeostasis of the holobiont is one of the objectives in pharmacological therapy, in order to implement healing strategies (Sarto-Jackson, 2018).

5.3 Ribosomes, secondary metabolism, and molecular evolution

To talk about the molecular evolution of secondary metabolism is to talk about the defense of space and adaptation and how it was crucial in the RNA world for the development of new multifunctional enzymes capable of catalyzing different processes and establishing metabolic networks (Andres, Blomeier, & Zurbriggen, 2019; Chevin & Beckerman, 2012). In this way, ribosomes played a fundamental role in the evolution of biosynthetic pathways for small molecules to acquire chemical diversity and biological function; that is, biosynthetic plasticity was a game of catalysis and storage of information (Asai et al., 2015; Braakman & Smith, 2013; Fischbach, Walsh, & Clardy, 2008). Now, when examining the role of secondary metabolism in biotic evolution, the presence and diversity of these in microorganisms can be explained as a source of fitness and their participation in eco-evolution, as is the case with *Streptomyces* species (Amara, Takano, & Breitling, 2018; Firn & Jones, 2000).

It has also been shown that the manipulation of ribosomal units induces changes in the production of compounds within microbial cells, which gives a potential application and innovation to this phenomenon of coevolution (Liu et al., 2018; Wang et al., 2018). However, ribosomes fulfill their greatest innovation by increasing the functionality of bioactive molecules in response to the chemical signals emitted during environmental changes (Erbas-Cakmak, Leigh, McTernan, & Nussbaumer, 2015; Monciardini, Iorio, Maffioli, Sosio, & Donadio, 2014). This fact consists in the ability of the ribosomes to regulate the expression of the enzymes responsible for biosynthesis, as well as the possibility of responding to chemical signals by changing the configuration of the enzymes produced, such as in the stringent response to the decrease in nutrients (Brown, Fernández, Gordiyenko, & Ramakrishnan, 2016; Zhou, Liao, Liao, Liao, & Lu, 2015).

It has also been demonstrated in microorganisms how the ribosome controlled stringent response induces the production of secondary metabolites (Kallifidas, Jiang, Ding, & Luesch, 2018; Wang et al., 2017). In addition, the microbial stringent response activates the chemical signals of quorum sensing and the induction of silent BGCs, giving it activity in regulation and modulation of adaptive responses (Irving & Corrigan, 2018; Van Delden, Comte, & Bally, 2001; Van der Meij, Worsley, Hutchings, & van Wezel, 2017). Likewise, stringent control is present in plants mediated by alarmone guanosine 5′-diphosphate 3′-diphosphate (ppGpp) and also induces the production of secondary metabolites under stress conditions (Stael et al., 2011). So this evolutionary mechanism linked to the ribosomes has allowed the variation of biosynthetic pathways in microorganisms; allowing the development of alternate routes of obtaining energy and new bioactive molecules, as well as being an important factor of resistance to antibiotics (Kanjee et al., 2011; Kim et al., 2013). So the study of this response of functional molecular evolution in the symbiosis can give advances in the design of microbial cell factories as well as the development of new antimicrobials with novel mechanisms of action.

5.4 Metabolomics in the holobiontic unit

One of the crucial factors to understand the autopoietic dynamics of the symbiosis and its metabolites is the study of the metabolomics of the holobiont as an evolutionary unit, because this is an expression of its metabolic pathways and adaptations for survival (Chaston & Douglas, 2012; Sogin, Putnam, Nelson, Anderson, & Gates, 2017). So in this way, the metabolomics of the symbiotic holobiont expresses the exchange of information, as well as the possible modifications of the hologenome in response to environmental changes (Farag et al., 2018). It is also important to bear in mind that the metabolites produced in symbiotic relationships have the function of inducing metabolic adaptations, as well as proliferation and movement in search of nutrient sources (Lyon, 2015; Smith-Ferguson & Beekman, 2019). Thus, in the symbiosis, the nucleotides that function as second messengers (cyclic AMP and cyclic GMP), and minerals like calcium, must fluctuate according to the established interactions (Mishra, Rastogi, & Shukla, 2012; Schue et al., 2011). In addition, in this mutualism the metabolism of lipids is modified to develop chemical signaling pathways with which to establish metabolic networks (Lastovetsky et al., 2016; Yu et al., 2011). Likewise, adaptive modifications of the expression of enzymes that catalyze biosynthetic pathways induce changes in protein synthesis and search for amino acid sources (van der Knaap & Verrijzer, 2016; Yuan, Sheppard, & Söll, 2008).

On the other hand metabolomic analysis in the holobiontic units show the effect that the microbiota exerts on the production of the metabolites, as well as in the modifications within the hologenome that produce genetic alterations in the holobiont, which opens the doors to a manipulation of the hologenome, configuring a new approach: pawnobiome (Theis et al., 2016; Voss, Leon, Dhurandhar, & Robb, 2015). Likewise, the nutritional conditions alter the conditions of the symbiotic relationships that can be observed in the metabolomic profiles as well as in the marked expression of groups of genes (Cleary, Condren, Zink, & Sanchez, 2017). Therefore, the study of holobiont metabolomes must consider the different environmental conditions that regulate them in order to establish the true nature of the symbioses involved (Calcott, Ackerley, Knight, Keyzers, & Owen, 2018; Sergaki, Lagunas, Lidbury, Gifford, & Schäfer, 2018). In addition, the hologenome metabolomics can show the chemical signaling mechanisms that induce evolution and mutation and allow fitness acquisition by the holobiont, as well as configuring the metagenome (Koskella, Hall, & Metcalf, 2017; Rosenberg & Zilber-Rosenberg, 2013). Thus, the correlation between metabolomics, metagenomics, and chemical evolution will give us the necessary information to establish the characteristics of biological synthesis systems that involve BGCs, biosynthetic enzymes, and posttranslational regulation carried out on ribosomes, as well as the role of cytochromes in the chemical diversity of symbiotic interactions (Eyles, Vior, & Truman, 2018; Sekurova, Schneider, & Zotchev, 2019; Ziemert, Alanjary, & Weber, 2016).

5.5 Metagenomics in the symbiopoiesis of holobionts

In order to conceive the adaptive changes in the hologenome mediated by the secondary metabolites, it is necessary to correlate the metagenomic information with the symbiosis of the holobiontic unit and thus understand the vertical transmission of the genetic information in the holobiont (Haag, 2018; Roughgarden, Gilbert, Rosenberg, Zilber-Rosenberg, & Lloyd, 2018). In this way, changes in the hologenome are acquired to the extent that they express a functionality that allows the biological system to adapt and survive, but each change induces modifications in the other holobionts of the system, thereby configuring a network of holobionts or metaholobionts, which share microorganisms, genetic resources and information (Osmanovic, Kessler, Rabin, & Soen, 2018; Vannier et al., 2019). Likewise, among the holobionts, there is sharing of chemical information corresponding to the signals produced by the secondary metabolism, with which a signaling network can be elucidated for coevolution (Hutzil, Sandoval-Motta, Frank, & Aldana, 2018; Lackner, Peters, Helfrich, & Piel, 2017).

Thus, obtaining the metagenomes present in symbiotic interactions is of fundamental importance to determine the organisms involved in the evolution of the holobiont, as well as to establish the BGCs that participate in the production of molecular communicators involved (Blair et al., 2018; Haque & Haque, 2017); this is in order to discover the biosynthetic potential of the metabolic networks that make up the evolutionary phenomenon of mutualism, in which molecular mediators express themselves in response to environmental stimuli affecting biological systems, and which can contribute to new pharmacological discoveries that allow the homeostasis of the holobiont (Harcombe, Chacón, Adamowicz, Chubiz, & Marx, 2018; Marchal et al., 2017). Likewise, describing the different chemical signals that take part in the metaholobiont will give the information to predict the biological activity of the molecules produced as well as their mechanisms of action and molecular targets (Shi & Bode, 2018). Finally, metagenomics is a source of information on the evolution of organisms in the environmental conditions where they have shaped their ecosystem; this fundamental factor makes important the bioprospecting of the various holobionts that inhabit the planet in order to determine their symbiotic relationships and innovations that they have developed in their mutualism (Hill & Sacristán-Soriano, 2017; Tinta et al., 2019).

5.6 Hologenome metabolomics: Adaptation in chemical diversity

When studying the molecular basis of the adaptation of the holobiont, which are encoded in the hologenome, and involve and connect all the information of the organisms belonging to the biological system, it is important to take into consideration all the present epigenetic factors that regulate resilience and plasticity (Salvucci, 2012). This is how epigenetic factors mediated by secondary metabolites help to regulate the adaptive response and expression of the hologenome inside the holobiont (Gundel, Rudgers, & Whitney, 2017; Macke, Tasiemski, Massol, Callens, & Decaestecker, 2017). Likewise, epigenetic modulators have chemical sensors that are inductors or repressors of expression, depending on environmental changes, as has been demonstrated with the components of the quorum sensing (Reis et al., 2016; You et al., 2006). In this way, the molecules that mediate the bacterial quorum sensing can induce the expression of host genes through the modulation of histones, thus demonstrating the capacity of the microbiota to stimulate adaptive responses in the host (Lai, Tan, & Pavelka, 2019; Neuman, Debelius, Knight, & Koren, 2015). Likewise, the quorum sensing, in mediating the formation of biofilms, induces the expression of BGCs to activate biosynthetic pathways that produce other varieties of chemically diverse compounds (Karatan & Watnick, 2009; Mao, Bushin, Moon, Wu, & Seyedsayamdost, 2017).

So these infochemicals, with which information is exchanged between organisms, are fundamental factors in the symbiosis and induction of mutation of the hologenomes (Dittami et al., 2019; Thompson, Rivera, Closek, & Medina, 2015). Additionally, the compounds that serve as molecular signals modify the hologenome to express the multifunctional enzymes required against the environmental changes what the microbiota sense (Bell et al., 2019; Jones, Kobayashi, Davies, Taga, & Walker, 2007). This is how the microbiome is part of the holobiont sensor system to collect information from the environment and produce chemical signals that alert the biological system to variations in ecosystems (Foster, Schluter, Coyte, & Rakoff-Nahoum, 2017; Mhlongo, Piater, Madala, Labuschagne, & Dubery, 2018). Equally, the chemical signals of the microbiome induce the expression of the silent BGCs to develop new biosynthetic pathways that allow access to nutrients and maintain energy flows in the biological system (Hug, Bader, Remškar, Cirnski, & Müller, 2018; Ongley, Bian, Neilan, & Müller, 2013). Likewise, the adaptation of the hologenome in interaction with the microbiome promotes the coevolution between both parties through the chemical symbiosis that they carry out (Fig. 3) (Brucker & Bordenstein, 2013; Ferreiro, Crook, Gasparrini, &

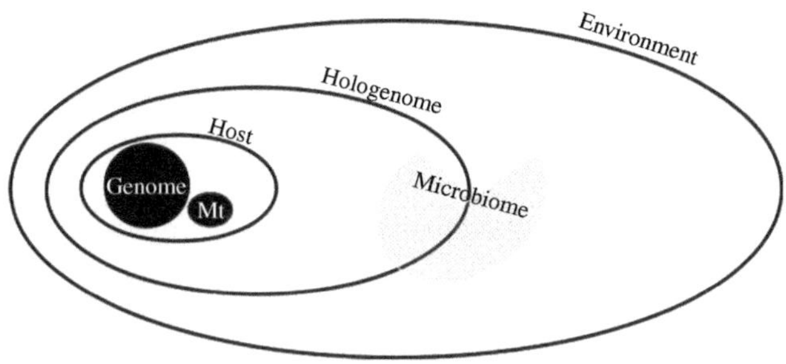

Fig. 3 Scheme of hologenome. Mt represents the mitochondria.

Dantas, 2018). Thus, the analysis of the chemical symbiosis modeled by the hologenomes will be a tool of great importance for the development of new biotechnological cell factories that will allow us to obtain new medicines with innovative mechanisms of action (Lee, Mattanovich, & Villaverde, 2012).

5.7 Symbiopoiesis and cognition: Life has commitment, concentration, and will

Life acquires cognition and self-reference of the world that surrounds it through secondary metabolism; this identifies the capacity of biological systems to interpret the environment and modulate their interaction (Brier, 2013; Pusztahelyi, Holb, & Pócsi, 2015). Thus, cognition is an organized system of chemical information that establishes a network in thermodynamic equilibrium that self-regulates (Kirchhoff, 2018; Vernon, Lowe, Thill, & Ziemke, 2015). In this way, bioactive molecules belong to a frame of reference for the search for homeostasis in the holobiont by inducing changes and response (Miller Jr., Torday, & Baluška, 2019). This network of chemical signals only evolves and acquires fitness to the extent that it interacts with the other members of the metaorganism (Röttjers & Faust, 2018). In this symbiotic concept, biological systems are open and not closed and acquire autopoiesis in conjunction with the entire biological community to which they belong in mutualism (Ruiz-Mirazo & Moreno, 2012). Thus, chemical mutualism is the key to establishing the metabolic networks with which to make the self-sustaining biological system within the holobiont (Root-Bernstein & Root-Bernstein, 2016). Thus, within the exchange of information, biological systems become more complex and their fitness capacity increases (Gilbert, Sapp, & Tauber, 2012). Finally, life is manifested in sharing and solidarity, as well as recognition within functionality.

5.8 Conclusions

The symbiosis in the mutualism configures the metabolic networks in the holobiont, which lead to the establishment of a homeostasis of the biological systems in coevolution (Shapira, 2016). In this way, the establishment of a secondary metabolism that produces biologically active compounds with which to communicate molecular information was a key factor in the acquisition of fitness (Roze, Chanda, & Linz, 2011). In addition, this molecular signaling has the ability to induce adaptation and mutation in the hologenome by inducing expression and modulation of genes related to biosynthesis (Moné, Monnin, & Kremer, 2014). In this way, when life acquired the capacity to synthesize bioactive molecules with which it communicated with the other organisms of the biological system, it was able to enter into symbiosis and mutualism within the ecosystems (Hunter, 2006). This enabled the holobiont to enter a framework of self-reference and cognition in molecular evolution. Thus, we can consider that a pharmacological treatment is the use of chemical signals that induce changes in the holobiont so that it can continue adapting to its environment (Rosenberg & Zilber-Rosenberg, 2018).

References

Amara, A., Takano, E., & Breitling, R. (2018). Development and validation of an updated computational model of Streptomyces coelicolor primary and secondary metabolism. *BMC Genomics*, *19*(1), 519.

Andres, J., Blomeier, T., & Zurbriggen, M. D. (2019). Synthetic switches and regulatory circuits in plants. *Plant Physiology*, *179*(3), 862–884.

Asai, T., Tsukada, K., Ise, S., Shirata, N., Hashimoto, M., Fujii, I., … Oshima, Y. (2015). Use of a biosynthetic intermediate to explore the chemical diversity of pseudo-natural fungal polyketides. *Nature Chemistry*, 7(9), 737.

Bang, C., Dagan, T., Deines, P., Dubilier, N., Duschl, W. J., Fraune, S., … Picazo, D. (2018). Metaorganisms in extreme environments: Do microbes play a role in organismal adaptation? *Zoology*, *127*, 1–19.

Bell, T. H., Hockett, K. L., Alcalá-Briseño, R. I., Barbercheck, M., Beattie, G. A., Bruns, M. A., … Esker, P. (2019). Manipulating wild and tamed phytobiomes: Challenges and opportunities. *Phytobiomes Journal*, *3*(1), 3–21.

Blair, P. M., Land, M. L., Piatek, M. J., Jacobson, D. A., Lu, T. Y. S., Doktycz, M. J., & Pelletier, D. A. (2018). Exploration of the biosynthetic potential of the Populus microbiome. *mSystems*, *3*(5), e00045-18.

Boudouresque, C. F., Caumette, P., Bertrand, J. C., Normand, P., & Sime-Ngando, T. (2015). Systematic and evolution of microorganisms: General concepts. In J.-C. Bertrand, P. Caumette, P. Lebaron, R. Matheron, P. Normand, & T. Sime-Ngando (Eds.), *Environmental microbiology: Fundamentals and applications* (pp. 107–144). Dordrecht: Springer.

Braakman, R., & Smith, E. (2013). The compositional and evolutionary logic of metabolism. *Physical Biology*, *10*(1), 011001.

Brier, S. (2013). Cybersemiotics: A new foundation for transdisciplinary theory of information, cognition, meaningful communication and the interaction between nature and culture. *Integral Review: A Transdisciplinary & Transcultural Journal for New Thought, Research, & Praxis, 9*(2), 220–263.

Brown, A., Fernández, I. S., Gordiyenko, Y., & Ramakrishnan, V. (2016). Ribosome-dependent activation of stringent control. *Nature, 534*(7606), 277.

Brucker, R. M., & Bordenstein, S. R. (2013). The capacious hologenome. *Zoology, 116*(5), 260–261.

Bueno, J. (2018). Looking for the integrome, when metabolomics talk about the interactome. *Journal of Microbial & Biochemical Technology, 10*, e134.

Calcott, M. J., Ackerley, D. F., Knight, A., Keyzers, R. A., & Owen, J. G. (2018). Secondary metabolism in the lichen symbiosis. *Chemical Society Reviews, 47*(5), 1730–1760.

Cavaliere, M., Feng, S., Soyer, O. S., & Jiménez, J. I. (2017). Cooperation in microbial communities and their biotechnological applications. *Environmental Microbiology, 19*(8), 2949–2963.

Chaston, J., & Douglas, A. E. (2012). Making the most of "omics" for symbiosis research. *The Biological Bulletin, 223*(1), 21–29.

Chevin, L. M., & Beckerman, A. P. (2012). From adaptation to molecular evolution. *Heredity, 108*(4), 457.

Cleary, J. L., Condren, A. R., Zink, K. E., & Sanchez, L. M. (2017). Calling all hosts: Bacterial communication *in situ*. *Chem, 2*(3), 334–358.

Debernardi, M., & Serrelli, E. (2013). From bacteria to Saint Francis to Gaia in the symbiotic view of evolution. *Evolution, 6*(1), 1–13.

Dittami, S. M., Arboleda, E., Auguet, J. C., Bigalke, A., Briand, E., Cárdenas, P., ... Gachon, C. M. (2019). *A community perspective on the concept of marine holobionts: State-of-the-art, challenges, and future directions (no. e27519v1)*. PeerJ Preprints.

Epstein, O. (2018). The spatial homeostasis hypothesis. *Symmetry, 10*(4), 103.

Erbas-Cakmak, S., Leigh, D. A., McTernan, C. T., & Nussbaumer, A. L. (2015). Artificial molecular machines. *Chemical Reviews, 115*(18), 10081–10206.

Etchegaray, J. P., & Mostoslavsky, R. (2016). Interplay between metabolism and epigenetics: A nuclear adaptation to environmental changes. *Molecular Cell, 62*(5), 695–711.

Eyles, T. H., Vior, N. M., & Truman, A. W. (2018). Rapid and robust yeast-mediated pathway refactoring generates multiple new bottromycin-related metabolites. *ACS Synthetic Biology*, 7(5), 1211–1218.

Farag, M. A., Meyer, A., Ali, S. E., Salem, M. A., Giavalisco, P., Westphal, H., & Wessjohann, L. A. (2018). Comparative metabolomics approach detects stress-specific responses during coral bleaching in soft corals. *Journal of Proteome Research, 17*(6), 2060–2071.

Ferreiro, A., Crook, N., Gasparrini, A. J., & Dantas, G. (2018). Multiscale evolutionary dynamics of host-associated microbiomes. *Cell, 172*(6), 1216–1227.

Firn, R. D., & Jones, C. G. (2000). The evolution of secondary metabolism–A unifying model. *Molecular Microbiology, 37*(5), 989–994.

Fischbach, M. A., Walsh, C. T., & Clardy, J. (2008). The evolution of gene collectives: How natural selection drives chemical innovation. *Proceedings of the National Academy of Sciences, 105*(12), 4601–4608.

Foster, K. R., Schluter, J., Coyte, K. Z., & Rakoff-Nahoum, S. (2017). The evolution of the host microbiome as an ecosystem on a leash. *Nature, 548*(7665), 43.

Fukui, S. (2014). Evolution of symbiosis with resource allocation from fecundity to survival. *Naturwissenschaften, 101*(5), 437–446.

Gilbert, S. F. (2014). Symbiosis as the way of eukaryotic life: The dependent co-origination of the body. *Journal of Biosciences, 39*(2), 201–209.

Gilbert, S. F., Sapp, J., & Tauber, A. I. (2012). A symbiotic view of life: We have never been individuals. *The Quarterly Review of Biology, 87*(4), 325–341.

Guerrero, R., & Berlanga, M. (2016). From the cell to the ecosystem: The physiological evolution of symbiosis. *Evolutionary Biology, 43*(4), 543–552.
Gundel, P. E., Rudgers, J. A., & Whitney, K. D. (2017). Vertically transmitted symbionts as mechanisms of transgenerational effects. *American Journal of Botany, 104*(5), 787–792.
Haag, K. L. (2018). Holobionts and their hologenomes: Evolution with mixed modes of inheritance. *Genetics and Molecular Biology, 41*(1 Suppl. 1), 189.
Haque, S. Z., & Haque, M. (2017). The ecological community of commensal, symbiotic, and pathogenic gastrointestinal microorganisms—An appraisal. *Clinical and Experimental Gastroenterology, 10*, 91.
Harcombe, W. R., Chacón, J. M., Adamowicz, E. M., Chubiz, L. M., & Marx, C. J. (2018). Evolution of bidirectional costly mutualism from byproduct consumption. *Proceedings of the National Academy of Sciences, 115*(47), 12000–12004.
Hill, M. S., & Sacristán-Soriano, O. (2017). Molecular and functional ecology of sponges and their microbial symbionts. In J. L. Carballo & J. J. James (Eds.), *Climate change, ocean acidification and sponges* (pp. 105–142). Cham: Springer.
Hug, J., Bader, C., Remškar, M., Cirnski, K., & Müller, R. (2018). Concepts and methods to access novel antibiotics from actinomycetes. *Antibiotics*, 7(2), 44.
Hunter, P. (2006). Entente cordiale: Multiple symbiosis illustrates the intricate interconnectivity of nature. *EMBO Reports*, 7(9), 861–864.
Hutzil, S., Sandoval-Motta, S., Frank, A., & Aldana, M. (2018). Modeling the role of the microbiome in evolution. *Frontiers in Physiology, 9*, 1836.
Irving, S. E., & Corrigan, R. M. (2018). Triggering the stringent response: Signals responsible for activating (p) ppGpp synthesis in bacteria. *Microbiology, 164*(3), 268–276.
Jones, K. M., Kobayashi, H., Davies, B. W., Taga, M. E., & Walker, G. C. (2007). How rhizobial symbionts invade plants: The Sinorhizobium–Medicago model. *Nature Reviews Microbiology, 5*(8), 619.
Kaessmann, H. (2010). Origins, evolution, and phenotypic impact of new genes. *Genome Research, 20*(10), 1313–1326.
Kallifidas, D., Jiang, G., Ding, Y., & Luesch, H. (2018). Rational engineering of Streptomyces albus J1074 for the overexpression of secondary metabolite gene clusters. *Microbial Cell Factories, 17*(1), 25.
Kanjee, U., Gutsche, I., Alexopoulos, E., Zhao, B., El Bakkouri, M., Thibault, G., … Houry, W. A. (2011). Linkage between the bacterial acid stress and stringent responses: The structure of the inducible lysine decarboxylase. *The EMBO Journal, 30*(5), 931–944.
Karatan, E., & Watnick, P. (2009). Signals, regulatory networks, and materials that build and break bacterial biofilms. *Microbiology and Molecular Biology Reviews, 73*(2), 310–347.
Kazamia, E., Helliwell, K. E., Purton, S., & Smith, A. G. (2016). How mutualisms arise in phytoplankton communities: Building eco-evolutionary principles for aquatic microbes. *Ecology Letters, 19*(7), 810–822.
Keller, N. P. (2018). Fungal secondary metabolism: Regulation, function and drug discovery. *Nature Reviews Microbiology, 17*, 167–180.
Kim, C., Mwangi, M., Chung, M., Milheirço, C., de Lencastre, H., & Tomasz, A. (2013). The mechanism of heterogeneous beta-lactam resistance in MRSA: Key role of the stringent stress response. *PLoS One, 8*(12), e82814.
Kirchhoff, M. D. (2018). Autopoiesis, free energy, and the life–mind continuity thesis. *Synthese, 195*(6), 2519–2540.
Koskella, B., Hall, L. J., & Metcalf, C. J. E. (2017). The microbiome beyond the horizon of ecological and evolutionary theory. *Nature Ecology & Evolution, 1*(11), 1606.
Lackner, G., Peters, E. E., Helfrich, E. J., & Piel, J. (2017). Insights into the lifestyle of uncultured bacterial natural product factories associated with marine sponges. *Proceedings of the National Academy of Sciences, 114*(3), E347–E356.

Lai, G. C., Tan, T. G., & Pavelka, N. (2019). The mammalian mycobiome: A complex system in a dynamic relationship with the host. *Wiley Interdisciplinary Reviews: Systems Biology and Medicine, 11*(1), e1438.
Lastovetsky, O. A., Gaspar, M. L., Mondo, S. J., LaButti, K. M., Sandor, L., Grigoriev, I.V., … Pawlowska, T. E. (2016). Lipid metabolic changes in an early divergent fungus govern the establishment of a mutualistic symbiosis with endobacteria. *Proceedings of the National Academy of Sciences, 113*(52), 15102–15107.
Lee, S.Y., Mattanovich, D., & Villaverde, A. (2012). Systems metabolic engineering, industrial biotechnology and microbial cell factories. *Microbial Cell Factories, 11*, 156.
Leigh, E. G., Jr. (2010). The evolution of mutualism. *Journal of Evolutionary Biology, 23*(12), 2507–2528.
Leitão, A. L., & Enguita, F. J. (2014). Fungal extrolites as a new source for therapeutic compounds and as building blocks for applications in synthetic biology. *Microbiological Research, 169*(9–10), 652–665.
Liu, L., Pan, J., Wang, Z., Yan, X., Yang, D., Zhu, X., … Huang, Y. (2018). Ribosome engineering and fermentation optimization leads to overproduction of tiancimycin A, a new enediyne natural product from *Streptomyces* sp. CB03234. *Journal of Industrial Microbiology & Biotechnology, 45*(3), 141–151.
Lucia, U. (2015). Bioengineering thermodynamics of biological cells. *Theoretical Biology and Medical Modelling, 12*(1), 29.
Lynch, M., Field, M. C., Goodson, H.V., Malik, H. S., Pereira-Leal, J. B., Roos, D. S., … Sazer, S. (2014). Evolutionary cell biology: Two origins, one objective. *Proceedings of the National Academy of Sciences, 111*(48), 16990–16994.
Lyon, P. (2015). The cognitive cell: Bacterial behavior reconsidered. *Frontiers in Microbiology, 6*, 264.
Macke, E., Tasiemski, A., Massol, F., Callens, M., & Decaestecker, E. (2017). Life history and eco-evolutionary dynamics in light of the gut microbiota. *Oikos, 126*(4), 508–531.
Mao, D., Bushin, L. B., Moon, K., Wu, Y., & Seyedsayamdost, M. R. (2017). Discovery of scmR as a global regulator of secondary metabolism and virulence in Burkholderia thailandensis E264. *Proceedings of the National Academy of Sciences, 114*(14), E2920–E2928.
Marchal, M., Goldschmidt, F., Derksen-Müller, S. N., Panke, S., Ackermann, M., & Johnson, D. R. (2017). A passive mutualistic interaction promotes the evolution of spatial structure within microbial populations. *BMC Evolutionary Biology, 17*(1), 106.
Mhlongo, M. I., Piater, L. A., Madala, N. E., Labuschagne, N., & Dubery, I. A. (2018). The chemistry of plant–microbe interactions in the rhizosphere and the potential for metabolomics to reveal signaling related to defense priming and induced systemic resistance. *Frontiers in Plant Science, 9*, 112.
Miller, W. (2016). Cognition, information fields and hologenomic entanglement: Evolution in light and shadow. *Biology, 5*(2), 21.
Miller, W. B., Jr. (2018). Biological information systems: Evolution as cognition-based information management. *Progress in Biophysics and Molecular Biology, 134*, 1–26.
Miller, W. B., Jr., Torday, J., & Baluška, F. (2019). Biological evolution as defense of 'self'. *Progress in Biophysics and Molecular Biology, 142*, 54–74.
Mishra, B. K., Rastogi, A., & Shukla, S. (2012). Regulatory role of mineral elements in the metabolism of medicinal plants. Mineral nutrition of medicinal and aromatic plants. *Medicinal and Aromatic Plant Science and Biotechnology, 6*, 1–23.
Monciardini, P., Iorio, M., Maffioli, S., Sosio, M., & Donadio, S. (2014). Discovering new bioactive molecules from microbial sources. *Microbial Biotechnology*, 7(3), 209–220.
Moné, Y., Monnin, D., & Kremer, N. (2014). The oxidative environment: A mediator of interspecies communication that drives symbiosis evolution. *Proceedings of the Royal Society B: Biological Sciences, 281*(1785), 20133112.

Muraille, E. (2018). Diversity generator mechanisms are essential components of biological systems: The two queen hypothesis. *Frontiers in Microbiology*, *9*, 223.

Neuman, H., Debelius, J. W., Knight, R., & Koren, O. (2015). Microbial endocrinology: The interplay between the microbiota and the endocrine system. *FEMS Microbiology Reviews*, *39*(4), 509–521.

Ongley, S. E., Bian, X., Neilan, B. A., & Müller, R. (2013). Recent advances in the heterologous expression of microbial natural product biosynthetic pathways. *Natural Product Reports*, *30*(8), 1121–1138.

Osmanovic, D., Kessler, D. A., Rabin, Y., & Soen, Y. (2018). Darwinian selection of host and bacteria supports emergence of Lamarckian-like adaptation of the system as a whole. *Biology Direct*, *13*(1), 24.

Pusztahelyi, T., Holb, I. J., & Pócsi, I. (2015). Secondary metabolites in fungus-plant interactions. *Frontiers in Plant Science*, *6*, 573.

Quin, M. B., Flynn, C. M., & Schmidt-Dannert, C. (2014). Traversing the fungal terpenome. *Natural Product Reports*, *31*(10), 1449–1473.

Razeto-Barry, P. (2012). Autopoiesis 40 years later. A review and a reformulation. *Origins of Life and Evolution of Biospheres*, *42*(6), 543–567.

Reis, S. A., Ghosh, B., Hendricks, J. A., Szantai-Kis, D. M., Törk, L., Ross, K. N., … Salthouse, C. (2016). Light-controlled modulation of gene expression by chemical optoepigenetic probes. *Nature Chemical Biology*, *12*(5), 317.

Rizzo, C., & Lo Giudice, A. (2018). Marine invertebrates: Underexplored sources of bacteria producing biologically active molecules. *Diversity*, *10*(3), 52.

Root-Bernstein, R., & Root-Bernstein, M. (2016). From compositional chemical ecologies to self-replicating ribosomes and on to functional trait ecological networks. In P. Pontarotti (Ed.), *Evolutionary biology* (pp. 327–343). Cham: Springer.

Rosenberg, E., & Zilber-Rosenberg, I. (2013). Microbiotas are part of holobiont fitness. In E. Rosenberg & I. Rosenberg (Eds.), *The hologenome concept: Human, animal and plant microbiota* (pp. 55–80). Cham: Springer.

Rosenberg, E., & Zilber-Rosenberg, I. (2018). The hologenome concept of evolution after 10 years. *Microbiome*, *6*(1), 78.

Röttjers, L., & Faust, K. (2018). From hairballs to hypotheses–biological insights from microbial networks. *FEMS Microbiology Reviews*, *42*(6), 761–780.

Roughgarden, J., Gilbert, S. F., Rosenberg, E., Zilber-Rosenberg, I., & Lloyd, E. A. (2018). Holobionts as units of selection and a model of their population dynamics and evolution. *Biological Theory*, *13*(1), 44–65.

Roze, L. V., Chanda, A., & Linz, J. E. (2011). Compartmentalization and molecular traffic in secondary metabolism: A new understanding of established cellular processes. *Fungal Genetics and Biology*, *48*(1), 35–48.

Ruiz-Mirazo, K., & Moreno, A. (2012). Autonomy in evolution: From minimal to complex life. *Synthese*, *185*(1), 21–52.

Salvucci, E. J. (2012). Selfishness, warfare, and economics; or integration, cooperation, and biology. *Frontiers in Cellular and Infection Microbiology*, *2*, 54.

Sarto-Jackson, I. (2018). Time for a change: Topical amendments to the medical model of disease. *Biological Theory*, *13*(1), 29–38.

Schmidt, E. W. (2015). The secret to a successful relationship: Lasting chemistry between ascidians and their symbiotic bacteria. *Invertebrate Biology*, *134*(1), 88–102.

Schmidt, E. W., Donia, M. S., McIntosh, J. A., Fricke, W. F., & Ravel, J. (2012). Origin and variation of tunicate secondary metabolites. *Journal of Natural Products*, *75*(2), 295–304.

Schue, M., Fekete, A., Ortet, P., Brutesco, C., Heulin, T., Schmitt-Kopplin, P., … Santaella, C. (2011). Modulation of metabolism and switching to biofilm prevail over exopolysaccharide production in the response of Rhizobium alamii to cadmium. *PLoS One*, *6*(11), e26771.

Sekurova, O. N., Schneider, O., & Zotchev, S. B. (2019). Novel bioactive natural products from bacteria via bioprospecting, genome mining and metabolic engineering. *Microbial Biotechnology*, *12*(5), 828–844.
Sergaki, C., Lagunas, B., Lidbury, I., Gifford, M. L., & Schäfer, P. (2018). Challenges and approaches in microbiome research: From fundamental to applied. *Frontiers in Plant Science*, *9*, 1205.
Shapira, M. (2016). Gut microbiotas and host evolution: Scaling up symbiosis. *Trends in Ecology & Evolution*, *31*(7), 539–549.
Shi, Y. M., & Bode, H. B. (2018). Chemical language and warfare of bacterial natural products in bacteria–nematode–insect interactions. *Natural Product Reports*, *35*(4), 309–335.
Smith-Ferguson, J., & Beekman, M. (2019). Who needs a brain? Slime moulds, behavioural ecology and minimal cognition. *Adaptive Behavior*, https://doi.org/10.1177/1059712319826537.
Sogin, E. M., Putnam, H. M., Nelson, C. E., Anderson, P., & Gates, R. D. (2017). Correspondence of coral holobiont metabolome with symbiotic bacteria, archaea and Symbiodinium communities. *Environmental Microbiology Reports*, *9*(3), 310–315.
Stael, S., Wurzinger, B., Mair, A., Mehlmer, N., Vothknecht, U. C., & Teige, M. (2011). Plant organellar calcium signalling: An emerging field. *Journal of Experimental Botany*, *63*(4), 1525–1542.
Steinberg, C. E., Stürzenbaum, S. R., & Menzel, R. (2008). Genes and environment—Striking the fine balance between sophisticated biomonitoring and true functional environmental genomics. *Science of the Total Environment*, *400*(1–3), 142–161.
Stringlis, I. A., Zhang, H., Pieterse, C. M., Bolton, M. D., & de Jonge, R. (2018). Microbial small molecules—Weapons of plant subversion. *Natural Product Reports*, *35*(5), 410–433.
Suárez, J. (2018). The importance of symbiosis in philosophy of biology: An analysis of the current debate on biological individuality and its historical roots. *Symbiosis*, *76*, 77–96.
Sudakaran, S., Kost, C., & Kaltenpoth, M. (2017). Symbiont acquisition and replacement as a source of ecological innovation. *Trends in Microbiology*, *25*(5), 375–390.
Terra, L. A., & Passador, J. L. (2016). Symbiotic dynamic: The strategic problem from the perspective of complexity. *Systems Research and Behavioral Science*, *33*(2), 235–248.
Theis, K. R., Dheilly, N. M., Klassen, J. L., Brucker, R. M., Baines, J. F., Bosch, T. C., … Sapp, J. (2016). Getting the hologenome concept right: An eco-evolutionary framework for hosts and their microbiomes. *mSystems*, *1*(2), e00028-16.
Thompson, J. R., Rivera, H. E., Closek, C. J., & Medina, M. (2015). Microbes in the coral holobiont: Partners through evolution, development, and ecological interactions. *Frontiers in Cellular and Infection Microbiology*, *4*, 176.
Tianero, M. D. B., Kwan, J. C., Wyche, T. P., Presson, A. P., Koch, M., Barrows, L. R., … Schmidt, E. W. (2015). Species specificity of symbiosis and secondary metabolism in ascidians. *The ISME Journal*, *9*(3), 615.
Tinta, T., Kogovšek, T., Klun, K., Malej, A., Herndl, G. J., & Turk, V. (2019). Jellyfish-associated microbiome in the marine environment: Exploring its biotechnological potential. *Marine Drugs*, *17*(2), 94.
Tu, Y., & Rappel, W. J. (2018). Adaptation in living systems. *Annual Review of Condensed Matter Physics*, *9*, 183–205.
Van Delden, C., Comte, R., & Bally, M. (2001). Stringent response activates quorum sensing and modulates cell density-dependent gene expression in Pseudomonas aeruginosa. *Journal of Bacteriology*, *183*(18), 5376–5384.
van der Knaap, J. A., & Verrijzer, C. P. (2016). Undercover: Gene control by metabolites and metabolic enzymes. *Genes & Development*, *30*(21), 2345–2369.
Van der Meij, A., Worsley, S. F., Hutchings, M. I., & van Wezel, G. P. (2017). Chemical ecology of antibiotic production by actinomycetes. *FEMS Microbiology Reviews*, *41*(3), 392–416.

Vannier, N., Mony, C., Bittebiere, A. K., Theis, K. R., Rosenberg, E., & Vandenkoornhuyse, P. (2019). Clonal plants as meta-holobionts. *mSystems*, *4*(2), e00213–e00218.
Vergara, R. C., Jaramillo-Riveri, S., Luarte, A., Moënne-Loccoz, C., Fuentes, R., Couve, A., & Maldonado, P. E. (2019). The energy homeostasis principle: Neuronal energy regulation drives local network dynamics generating behavior. *Frontiers in Computational Neuroscience*, *13*, 49.
Vernon, D., Lowe, R., Thill, S., & Ziemke, T. (2015). Embodied cognition and circular causality: On the role of constitutive autonomy in the reciprocal coupling of perception and action. *Frontiers in Psychology*, *6*, 1660.
Vitas, M., & Dobovišek, A. (2018). In the beginning was a mutualism-on the origin of translation. *Origins of Life and Evolution of Biospheres*, *48*, 223–243.
Voss, J. D., Leon, J. C., Dhurandhar, N.V., & Robb, F.T. (2015). Pawnobiome: Manipulation of the hologenome within one host generation and beyond. *Frontiers in Microbiology*, *6*, 697.
Wang, L., Li, S., Zhao, J., Liu, Y., Chen, X., Tang, L., & Mao, Z. (2018). Efficiently activated ε-poly-L-lysine production by multiple antibiotic-resistance mutations and acidic pH shock optimization in Streptomyces albulus. *MicrobiologyOpen*, *8*, e00728.
Wang, J., Liu, H., Huang, D., Jin, L., Wang, C., & Wen, J. (2017). Comparative proteomic and metabolomic analysis of Streptomyces tsukubaensis reveals the metabolic mechanism of FK506 overproduction by feeding soybean oil. *Applied Microbiology and Biotechnology*, *101*(6), 2447–2465.
Wang, R., & Seyedsayamdost, M. R. (2017). Opinion: Hijacking exogenous signals to generate new secondary metabolites during symbiotic interactions. *Nature Reviews Chemistry*, *1*(3), 0021.
Wichard, T., & Beemelmanns, C. (2018). Role of chemical mediators in aquatic interactions across the prokaryote–eukaryote boundary. *Journal of Chemical Ecology*, *44*(11), 1008–1021.
Wisecaver, J. H., Borowsky, A. T., Tzin, V., Jander, G., Kliebenstein, D. J., & Rokas, A. (2017). A global coexpression network approach for connecting genes to specialized metabolic pathways in plants. *The Plant Cell*, *29*(5), 944–959.
You, Y. S., Marella, H., Zentella, R., Zhou, Y., Ulmasov, T., Ho, T. H. D., & Quatrano, R. S. (2006). Use of bacterial quorum-sensing components to regulate gene expression in plants. *Plant Physiology*, *140*(4), 1205–1212.
Yu, W. L., Ansari, W., Schoepp, N. G., Hannon, M. J., Mayfield, S. P., & Burkart, M. D. (2011). Modifications of the metabolic pathways of lipid and triacylglycerol production in microalgae. *Microbial Cell Factories*, *10*(1), 91.
Yuan, J., Sheppard, K., & Söll, D. (2008). Amino acid modifications on tRNA. *Acta Biochimica et Biophysica Sinica*, *40*(7), 539–553.
Zhou, X., Liao, W. J., Liao, J. M., Liao, P., & Lu, H. (2015). Ribosomal proteins: Functions beyond the ribosome. *Journal of Molecular Cell Biology*, *7*(2), 92–104.
Ziemert, N., Alanjary, M., & Weber, T. (2016). The evolution of genome mining in microbes—A review. *Natural Product Reports*, *33*(8), 988–1005.

CHAPTER 6

Metabolomics of epigenetics: A history of the integrome

The scientist is not a person who gives the right answers, he's one who asks the right questions.

Claude Levi-Strauss (1908–2009)

It necessarily follows that chance alone is at the source of every innovation, and of all creation in the biosphere. Pure chance, absolutely free but blind, at the very root of the stupendous edifice of evolution: this central concept of modern biology is no longer one among many other possible or even conceivable hypotheses. It is today the sole conceivable hypothesis, the only one that squares with observed and tested fact. And nothing warrants the supposition - or the hope - that on this score our position is ever likely to be revised. There is no scientific concept, in any of the sciences, more destructive of anthropocentrism than this one.

Jacques Monod (1910–76)

6.1 Introduction

When trying to address the question about the secondary metabolites that mediate epigenetic regulation, inducing or repressing the expression of special genes for obtaining nutrients and communication, it is necessary to unite several approaches, one of which is metabolomics (Qadri et al., 2017). Thus, the presence and synthesis in the symbiotic interactions of small-molecule epigenetic modifiers allows the metabolic network to remain in equilibrium for the benefit of the holobiont (Asgari, 2014; Betts et al., 2014; Thomas et al., 2009). Then the symbiosis is enriched to the extent that a greater number of epigenetic modifiers are produced to increase molecular communication within the biological system (Egan, Loscri, Duong, & Di Renzo, 2019; Mazzio & Soliman, 2014). Similarly, in this mutualism, the reversible and sustainable chemical modification of the histones surrounding the DNA is among the most involved epigenetic

Molecular Evolutionary Models in Drug Discovery
https://doi.org/10.1016/B978-0-12-817613-9.00006-7

phenomena (Meyer, 2015; Tammen, Friso, & Choi, 2013). This chemical regulation of the function of histones to modulate gene expression in response to environmental changes has been the basis of molecular evolution by changing the enzymes that make the synthesis, which leads to the emergence of new biosynthetic pathways and by, consequently, greater diversity (Etchegaray & Mostoslavsky, 2016; Metallo & Vander Heiden, 2013; Schvartzman, Thompson, & Finley, 2018). Equally, histone posttranslational modifications (PTMs) have the capacity to respond to nutritional and environmental changes, as well as hormone-mediated stimulation, using the following mechanisms (Fig. 1) (Conaway, 2018; Fan, Krautkramer, Feldman, & Denu, 2015):

- acetylation of lysine or N-termini;
- methylation of lysine and arginine;
- phosphorylation of serine threonine and tyrosine;
- fatty acylation; and
- ADP-ribosylation.

Thus, the analysis of the metabolic fluxes of the epigenetic modifications is a key piece for the understanding of the symbiosis in the holobiont, as well as its autopoiesis and hologenomic evolution (Hurst, 2017; Paniagua Voirol, Frago, Kaltenpoth, Hilker, & Fatouros, 2018). In addition, it is important to integrate the omics disciplines around the study of the mutualistic interactions that make up the complex biological systems around the search for an integrome that encompasses the connections and exchange of information, as well as the energy necessary for molecular evolution to have been carried out (Fig. 2) (Buescher & Driggers, 2016).

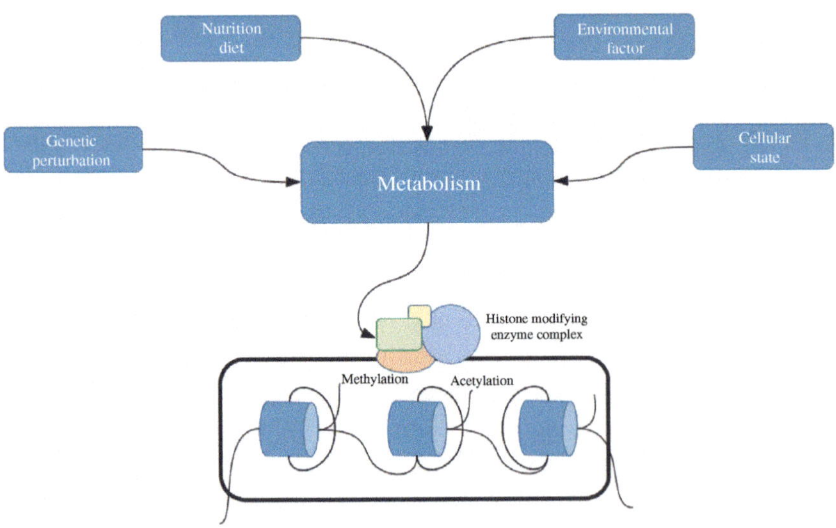

Fig. 1 Histone posttranslational modifications.

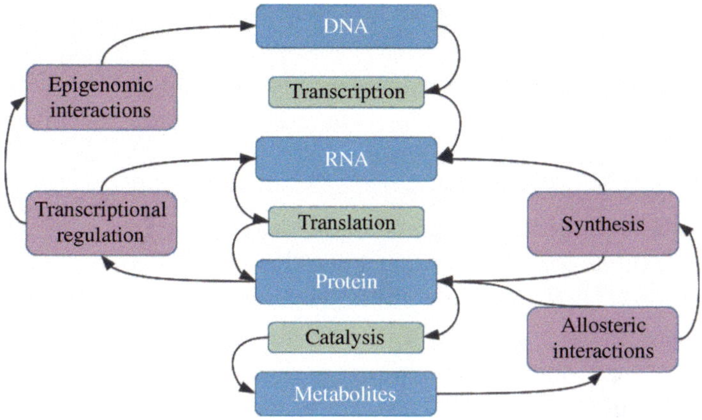

Fig. 2 The relationship among the -omics levels.

On the other hand, small molecules as epigenetic modifiers will allow the development of the design and development of new drugs and products capable of achieving homeostasis by regulating the epigenetic response in the holobiont, with which a new approach in medicine could be obtained (Runcie, Chan, Zengerle, & Ciulli, 2016; Xie, Zang, Li, & Shu, 2016). For this reason, the objective of this chapter is to analyze epigenetics as a source of chemical evolution and a fundamental part of metabolic networks that allow adaptation and fitness, as well as their therapeutic possibilities and perspectives (Burggren, 2016; Kanherkar, Bhatia-Dey, & Csoka, 2014).

6.2 Metabolic flux analysis of epigenetics: The route toward chemical diversity

The metabolic mechanisms of epigenetic regulation affect processes including histone acetylation, histone methylation, and DNA methylation (Meier, 2013). This is how secondary metabolites modulate the chemical modifications of histones that regulate gene expression (Nieborak & Schneider, 2018). Also among the metabolites to which the histones react are reactive oxygen species (ROS), which are produced in the mitochondria during the phenomena of cellular stress, this as part of a network that allows adaptation and fitness (Picard, McEwen, Epel, & Sandi, 2018; Son & Lee, 2019). Thus, in this way, the metabolic fluxes of epigenetics must be aimed at obtaining nutrients, responding to environmental stress, and establishing communication networks within the biological system, which translates into phenotypic robustness and plasticity (Nijhout, Sadre-Marandi, Best, & Reed,

2017; Torday & Miller, 2016). In this way, this epigenetically modulated phenotypic robustness and plasticity was acquired as a primitive response to oxidative stress, which allowed the evolution of the RNA world; a phenomenon that persists until today, where RNA molecules suffer and are susceptible to epigenetic modifications (Duncan, Gluckman, & Dearden, 2014; Frías-Lasserre & Villagra, 2017).

This is how the secondary metabolism was enriched by epigenetic modifications in RNA, establishing metabolic fluxes as the guide for adaptation and evolution (Cyr & Domann, 2011; Thiebaut, Hemerly, & Ferreira, 2019); equally, the epigenetic modifications impulse the evolution of biosynthetic pathways as they obtained functionality and complexity (Badyaev, 2014; Beldade, Mateus, & Keller, 2011). In this way, epigenetically modulated biosynthetic pathways acquired chemical diversity, through the functionality that their products and processes developed in response to an environment; this means that bioactive molecules are the result of adaptation prior to mutation (King, Edgar, Qiao, & Stephanopoulos, 2016; Strauss & Reyes-Dominguez, 2011). Furthermore, histone modifications induce a chemical diversity of chromatin that allows the expression of certain genes, and thus, the synthesis of varied enzymes that develop chemical innovations (Rothbart & Strahl, 2014; Law, Cheung, & Adhvaryu, 2015). Likewise, these chemically diverse molecules acting as signaling molecules also have the capacity to epigenetically modulate other cells in the biological system, which can establish a molecular communication network that allows the search for homeostasis and fitness (Chirumbolo & Bjørklund, 2017; Naviaux, 2018).

On the other hand, microbial communication systems such as quorum sensing can also mediate epigenetic modifications in the host cells and therefore in the hologenome (Greer, Dong, Morgun, & Shulzhenko, 2016; Westerhoff et al., 2014). This ability to exchange chemical signals and recognize them among different prokaryotic and eukaryotic species makes the holobiontic unit capable of interacting and making phenotypic changes in coevolution (Kutschera, 2018; Shapiro, 2017). Equally, the epigenetic phenomenon should be taken into account in the translation of proteins into ribosomes, especially in ribosomal DNA (rDNA), that codifies the RNA molecules present in the ribosomes and affecting their biogenesis; this phenomena modifies the enzymatic structure and makes the biosynthesis obtain various products with diverse biological functions (Byrgazov, Vesper, & Moll, 2013; Holland, 2017). In this way it has been reported that methylation of bacterial 16S rRNA is regulated epigenetically by quorum sensing molecules, as well as molecular induction of deacetylation of histones in genes that express ribosomal RNA in plants (Liu et al., 2014; Reigstad & Kashyap, 2013). Thus, the epigenetic modification of the enzymes allowed the biosynthetic pathways to increase their diversity and robustness as they responded to environmental changes and interacted with biological systems, resulting in a greater acquisition of complexity (Sneppen, 2017; Wang, Liu, & Sun, 2017). Finally, the diversity of the secondary metabolism was configured in the response to environmental factors and in its functionality became inheritable; that is the chance and the necessity (Bennett & Moran, 2015; Mushegian & Ebert, 2016).

6.3 Epigenetics in the RNA world: The rise of fitness

Methylation of RNA mediated by RNA methyltransferases (MTases) was prior to DNA methylation; this in order to protect the gene information, as well as the enzymatic activity that allowed fitness, obtaining of energy, and molecular communication (Rana & Ankri, 2016). In addition, the synthesis of small noncoding RNAs (sncRNAs) and long noncoding RNAs (lncRNAs) allowed the protocell to regulate its functional biology epigenetically (Hanly, Esteller, & Berdasco, 2018; Huang & Zhang, 2014). Likewise, ribosomal RNA is susceptible to being modified, constituting an epitranscriptomic model that drives the heterogeneity of biosynthetic pathways, as well as chemical diversity (Monaco, Marcel, Diaz, & Catez, 2018; Sergiev, Aleksashin, Chugunova, Polikanov, & Dontsova, 2018). In addition, the second messengers of RNA and riboswitches susceptible to AMP and GMP gave greater versatility to protein synthesis to achieve fitness in the original environment (Breaker, 2012; Mellin & Cossart, 2015; Nelson et al., 2013). Thus, homeostasis mediated by AMP and GMP allowed adaptation to stress through transcriptional regulation in the RNA world (Bastet, Dubé, Massé, & Lafontaine, 2011).

In this way, epigenetic regulation and protection in the RNA world by methylation had the ability to achieve the establishment of the metabolic networks necessary for the maintenance of catalytic activities, and also the osmotic homeostasis mediated by the second messengers maintained the conditions conducive to the development of the functional processes (Forman, Fukuto, & Torres, 2004; Ladurner, 2006). Originally, the thiol-rich peptides (TRPs) that were already present carried out both the catalytic processes and, in the development of epigenetic regulation in RNA, chemical processes that continue to this day (Shalayel, Coulibaly, Ly, Milet, & Vallée, 2018; Vallee et al., 2017). Equally, thiol-rich peptides (TRP) developed processes of posttranslational regulation of protein synthesis in the first ribosomes allowing the development of innovations in biosynthetic pathways (Müller, 2017; Noller, 2012). Thus, epigenetics and epitranscriptomics were fundamental tools for the RNA world to acquire fitness by being able to establish molecular communication networks that increased in complexity and openness the existing metabolic networks in the biological system (Jandura & Krause, 2017; Kun et al., 2015). That means more versatile synthesis routes with greater plasticity and chemical diversity capacity.

6.4 Multifunctional enzymes and epigenetic regulation: The source of promiscuity

Thanks to enzymatic promiscuity, the protocell was able to catalyze a large number of reactions and to metabolize more substrates, but this promiscuity was also the result of the phenotypic adaptations regulated by the epigenetics and epitranscriptomics (Chen, Salehi-Ashtiani, & Szostak, 2005; Roundtree, Evans, Pan, & He, 2017; Schaefer, Kapoor, & Jantsch, 2017). Likewise, by inducing modifications in RNA that lead to enzymatic promiscuity, biosynthetic pathways acquire innovation and produce greater diversity (Carbonell, Lecointre, & Faulon, 2011; Copley, 2015; Noda-Garcia, Liebermeister, & Tawfik, 2018). Furthermore, in the symbiosis, the greater number of biologically active metabolites assume greater functionality as more chemical information is exchanged and these characteristics are due to the susceptibility of the RNA to being modified (Lyon, 2017; Speijer, 2017). Likewise, in biosynthetic gene clusters (BGCs), the epigenetic regulation in gene expression increases enzymatic multifunctionality, achieving the production of a great variety of molecular communicators capable of establishing relations of mutualism within the holobiont (Brakhage, 2013; Pfannenstiel & Keller, 2019).

On the other hand, the production of secondary metabolites can be induced by the RNA polymerase (RNAP), which, through the bacterial linkage with bacterial alarmone ppGpp, can activate the expression of the BGCs (Ancona et al., 2015; Baral, Akhgari, & Metsä-Ketelä, 2018). In addition, in bacteria, the alarmone ppGpp, through the promotion of the production of multifunctional enzymes, regulates metabolism, growth, and stress tolerance (Kriel et al., 2012; Steinchen & Bange, 2016). Thus stress and its adaptive response are the source of the multifunctionality of enzymes, as well as the epigenetic and epitranscriptomic regulation that seeks homeostasis in the biological system (Clare, Brassington, Kwong, & Sinclair, 2019; Song & Yi, 2017; Thomas, Batista, & Meier, 2019). In addition, ncRNAs performs a transcriptional and posttranscriptional regulation that also leads to the assembly of enzymes with a high catalysis capacity, which gives greater robustness to metabolic networks (He, Fromion, & Westerhoff, 2013; Mohanty & Kushner, 2018). In this way, lncRNAs are the most closely associated with ribosomes and can induce chromatin modifications, as well as modulate DNA methylation, giving it a key role in the production of biosynthetic enzymes (Fatica & Bozzoni, 2014; Matzke, Kanno, & Matzke, 2015). Furthermore, in eukaryotes, the RNA-directed DNA methylation (RdDM) process is regulated by sncRNAs, inducing the production of secondary metabolites in fungi and plants (Contreras-Cubas, Palomar, Arteaga-Vázquez, Reyes, & Covarrubias, 2012; Moler et al., 2018). Equally, this mechanism responds to environmental factors such as light, thus promoting adaptive phenotypic changes that result in the production of functional secondary metabolic components (Kuo et al., 2015; Lelandais-Brière et al., 2010; Yaish, 2013).

Thus, secondary metabolites end up being the response to abiotic and biotic stress; response that is modulated from the epigenetic modifications becomes more varied as fitness is acquired (Gutzat & Scheid, 2012; Ramirez-Prado et al., 2018; Yaish, 2017). These responses consist of three phases; namely: first, molecular signaling, where compounds such as salicylic acid (SA) and jasmonic acid (JA) in plants act as environmental sensors that alert biological systems; second, involvement of the chromatin structure by processes such as histone acetylation and DNA methylation in response to chemical signals in order to regulate the expression of biosynthetic pathways in response to stress; finally, if the environmental factor persists there is an epigenetic response that reprograms reproduction and growth as it is stringently controlled (Mhlongo, Piater, Madala, Labuschagne, & Dubery, 2018; Sewelam, Kazan, & Schenk, 2016). So signaling and molecular alert of epigenetics leads to the mutualism of the holobiont between its symbionts and the host, where the environmental signals are transduced in a chemical way so that the hologenome enters an adaptive process that determines the coevolution (Renoz et al., 2017; Sorek et al., 2018; Thomas et al., 2017), and so enzymatic promiscuity was a key piece in the symbiosis that drove the evolution of metabolic replicators, as well as the establishment of metabolic networks (Braakman & Smith, 2012; Könnyű & Czárán, 2011).

6.5 Fluxomics, adaptomics, and epigenomics in the holobiontic unit

In this way the fluxomics determines the rate of metabolic reactions in a biological system. These metabolic interactions are regulated epigenetically in response to environmental stress by virtue of the adaptation and also configure the symbiosis present in the holobiont (Cortassa et al., 2015). Thus, the fluxomics of metabolite production by symbionts will have the ability to influence the epigenetic response of the host to modulate gene expression in the hologenome (Shen et al., 2012). So it can be concluded that symbionts chemically transduce environmental signals, epigenetically modulating the host, inducing adaptive changes of phenotypic type (Chiu & Gilbert, 2015; Shapiro, 2019). In addition, these symbionts represented by bacteria, archaebacteria, fungi, viruses, and parasites are in constant chemical exchange with the host inside the holobiont and regulate the functional responses to stress (Dheilly, 2014; van de Water, Allemand, & Ferrier-Pagès, 2018). This multispecies mutualism also promotes symbiotic adaptation for the acquisition of nutrients and constitution of metabolic networks to obtain the energy of the biological system (Hussa & Goodrich-Blair, 2013; Pradeu, 2016; Rowland et al., 2018).

In this way, signaling molecules, such as acyl homoserine lactone produced by bacteria during the phenomenon of quorum sensing, induce epigenetic regulation in the host (Churchill & Chen, 2010; Schuster, Joseph Sexton, Diggle, & Peter Greenberg, 2013). In addition, acyl homoserine lactone is produced by bacteria in response to stress to induce the formation of biofilms and make histone modifications, thus achieving expression of bioactive molecules that carry new chemical signals to the host (Schenk et al., 2014; Zarins-Tutt et al., 2016). Thus the set of metabolic reactions of a holobiont will be determined by the search for nutrients and the environmental factors of the ecosystem where it coexists, and all the phenotypic adaptations that the biological system requires for survival are the result of the connection between the metabolites and epigenetic regulation, in order to increase versatility and plasticity (Sandoval-Motta, Aldana, & Frank, 2017; Vorholt, Vogel, Carlström, & Mueller, 2017)

6.6 Inheritable symbiosis in adaptation

The ability to enter into interaction and communication as well as to establish metabolic networks must be heritable to allow survival through the generations; this is the key by which phenotypic adaptations can be passed to permanent genotypic changes (Ryall, Eydallin, & Ferenci, 2012; Wagner, 2012). In this way the epigenetic ability to acquire robustness to develop alternative metabolic pathways with which to obtain nutrients and communicate with other individuals of the biological system, as well as transduce environmental chemical signals to the host in a holobiont, are characteristics that are maintained through coevolution (Marijuán, Navarro, & del Moral, 2015, 2018). In this way, a macromolecular network for adaptation makes cognition and self-reference inherit among individuals in the biological system and is encoded in the hologenome (Westerhoff et al., 2014). So inheriting the robustness for adaptation—call this the search for nutrients and homeostasis—is inheriting the ability to learn; epigenetics provides that ability to learn (Heard & Martienssen, 2014; Norouzitallab, Baruah, Vanrompay, & Bossier, 2018). This ability to learn, provided by epigenetics, is manifested by moving from phenotypic adaptations to coding in the genome of functional changes acquired by the biological system for survival (Fox, Donelson, Schunter, Ravasi, & Gaitán-Espitia, 2019). So this possibility of learning in adaptation to environmental conditions arose from the susceptibility to different chemical signals and metabolites to induce changes in the expression of genetic information and thus obtain innovations translated into chemical diversity (Ehrenreich & Pfennig, 2015).

6.7 Epigenetics, epitranscriptomics, and the integrome: Adaptation in biotechnological innovation

Thus, epigenetic adaptations are key to the development of new products with utility in medicine, agriculture, and industry, because modifications in expression can modify metabolic pathways in response to environmental changes and induce chemical innovation (Etchegaray & Mostoslavsky, 2016; Miousse et al., 2015). In this way, the manipulation of the acetylation of histones and the methylation of DNA and RNA are fundamental tools to optimize the processes of obtaining biologically active molecules in biotechnological processes (Chen, Li, Subramaniam, Shyy, & Chien, 2017). One example of this possibility is the design and development of new DNA polymerases, whose modifications and heterogeneity derive in the production of new enzymes with an expanded spectrum of substrates (Aschenbrenner & Marx, 2017). Likewise, epigenetics opens up the pharmacological possibility of inducing the adaptation of the holobiont and the study of the biochemical functionality of its metabolic pathways (Crittenden & Schnorr, 2017). Additionally, the use of histone acetylation modulators to increase the production of secondary metabolites in biotechnological processes has proven to be a tool with great impact for obtaining new products (Chen, Smanski, & Shen, 2010; Santos, Pires, & Abranches, 2017).

The study of epitranscriptomics, especially in the modifications to ribosomal RNA, constitutes an important approach in the search for the development of new enzymes and the production of biologically active molecules by cracking the specific transcription processes involved (Bangru & Kalsotra, 2016). Equally, the use of acyl homoserine lactones as inducers of epigenetic regulation, as well as the expression of silent BGCs in bioreactors for the production of chemically diverse secondary metabolites, is a promising possibility (Reen, Romano, Dobson, & O'Gara, 2015). Finally, epigenetic nutrition deserves a separate mention, in which the use of probiotic and synbiotic products to make modifications of gene expression in the host can be an interesting therapeutic approach in the search for homeostasis in the holobiont (Markowiak & Śliżewska, 2018;Yang, Owen, Lightfoot, Kladde, & Mohamadzadeh, 2013).

6.8 Conclusions

Epigenetics in the control of secondary metabolism is a discipline of integration of metabolic networks with phenotypic adaptations (Fondi & Liò, 2015); thus, in this fitness acquisition, it is possible to produce chemically diverse metabolites that regulate a greater number of processes, as well as modified enzymes capable of metabolizing a broad spectrum of substrates (Adrio & Demain, 2014). In this way, the necessary integration of epigenomics and epitranscriptomics in a complex system that involves fluxomics in a study of adaptation or adaptomics will allow us to obtain a wide range of information on a biological phenomenon such as symbiosis and mutualism (Mazzio & Soliman, 2012), in order to obtain a frame of reference for health and disease within the holobiont, as well as how to acquire homeostasis within the biological system (Torday & Miller Jr., 2016). Likewise, the study of phenotypic adaptations is a source of tools and applications for the development of new processes with which to implement biotechnological innovations, as well as for the understanding of the cognitive mechanisms that are carried out within complex systems and allow them to achieve survival and persistence (Gluckman, Low, Buklijas, Hanson, & Beedle, 2011).

References

Adrio, J., & Demain, A. (2014). Microbial enzymes: Tools for biotechnological processes. *Biomolecules*, *4*(1), 117–139.

Ancona, V., Lee, J. H., Chatnaparat, T., Oh, J., Hong, J. I., & Zhao, Y. (2015). The bacterial alarmone (p) ppGpp activates the type III secretion system in *Erwinia amylovora*. *Journal of Bacteriology*, *197*(8), 1433–1443.

Aschenbrenner, J., & Marx, A. (2017). DNA polymerases and biotechnological applications. *Current Opinion in Biotechnology*, *48*, 187–195.
Asgari, S. (2014). Epigenetic modifications underlying symbiont–host interactions. *Advances in Genetics*, *86*, 253–276.
Badyaev, A.V. (2014). Epigenetic resolution of the 'curse of complexity'in adaptive evolution of complex traits. *The Journal of Physiology*, *592*(11), 2251–2260.
Bangru, S., & Kalsotra, A. (2016). Advances in analyzing RNA diversity in eukaryotic transcriptomes: Peering through the Omics lens. *F1000Research*, *5*, .
Baral, B., Akhgari, A., & Metsä-Ketelä, M. (2018). Activation of microbial secondary metabolic pathways: Avenues and challenges. *Synthetic and Systems Biotechnology*, *3*(3), 163.
Bastet, L., Dubé, A., Massé, E., & Lafontaine, D. A. (2011). New insights into riboswitch regulation mechanisms. *Molecular Microbiology*, *80*(5), 1148–1154.
Beldade, P., Mateus, A. R. A., & Keller, R. A. (2011). Evolution and molecular mechanisms of adaptive developmental plasticity. *Molecular Ecology*, *20*(7), 1347–1363.
Bennett, G. M., & Moran, N. A. (2015). Heritable symbiosis: The advantages and perils of an evolutionary rabbit hole. *Proceedings of the National Academy of Sciences*, *112*(33), 10169–10176.
Betts, M. J., Lu, Q., Jiang, Y., Drusko, A., Wichmann, O., Utz, M., … Pfister, S. (2014). Mechismo: Predicting the mechanistic impact of mutations and modifications on molecular interactions. *Nucleic Acids Research*, *43*(2), e10.
Braakman, R., & Smith, E. (2012). The compositional and evolutionary logic of metabolism. *Physical Biology*, *10*(1), 011001.
Brakhage, A. A. (2013). Regulation of fungal secondary metabolism. *Nature Reviews Microbiology*, *11*(1), 21.
Breaker, R. R. (2012). Riboswitches and the RNA world. *Cold Spring Harbor Perspectives in Biology*, *4*(2), a003566.
Buescher, J. M., & Driggers, E. M. (2016). Integration of omics: More than the sum of its parts. *Cancer & Metabolism*, *4*(1), 4.
Burggren, W. (2016). Epigenetic inheritance and its role in evolutionary biology: Re-evaluation and new perspectives. *Biology*, *5*(2), 24.
Byrgazov, K., Vesper, O., & Moll, I. (2013). Ribosome heterogeneity: Another level of complexity in bacterial translation regulation. *Current Opinion in Microbiology*, *16*(2), 133–139.
Carbonell, P., Lecointre, G., & Faulon, J. L. (2011). Origins of specificity and promiscuity in metabolic networks. *Journal of Biological Chemistry*, *286*(51), 43994–44004.
Chen, Z., Li, S., Subramaniam, S., Shyy, J. Y. J., & Chien, S. (2017). Epigenetic regulation: A new frontier for biomedical engineers. *Annual Review of Biomedical Engineering*, *19*, 195–219.
Chen, I. A., Salehi-Ashtiani, K., & Szostak, J. W. (2005). RNA catalysis in model protocell vesicles. *Journal of the American Chemical Society*, *127*(38), 13213–13219.
Chen, Y., Smanski, M. J., & Shen, B. (2010). Improvement of secondary metabolite production in Streptomyces by manipulating pathway regulation. *Applied Microbiology and Biotechnology*, *86*(1), 19–25.
Chirumbolo, S., & Bjørklund, G. (2017). PERM hypothesis: The fundamental machinery able to elucidate the role of xenobiotics and hormesis in cell survival and homeostasis. *International Journal of Molecular Sciences*, *18*(1), 165.
Chiu, L., & Gilbert, S. F. (2015). The birth of the holobiont: Multi-species birthing through mutual scaffolding and niche construction. *Biosemiotics*, *8*(2), 191–210.
Churchill, M. E., & Chen, L. (2010). Structural basis of acyl-homoserine lactone-dependent signaling. *Chemical Reviews*, *111*(1), 68–85.
Clare, C. E., Brassington, A. H., Kwong, W. Y., & Sinclair, K. D. (2019). One-carbon metabolism: Linking nutritional biochemistry to epigenetic programming of long-term development. *Annual Review of Animal Biosciences*, *7*, 263–287.

Conaway, R. C. (2018). Metabolic regulation of transcription and chromatin. *Annual Review of Biochemistry*, *87*, 23–25.

Contreras-Cubas, C., Palomar, M., Arteaga-Vázquez, M., Reyes, J. L., & Covarrubias, A. A. (2012). Non-coding RNAs in the plant response to abiotic stress. *Planta*, *236*(4), 943–958.

Copley, S. D. (2015). An evolutionary biochemist's perspective on promiscuity. *Trends in Biochemical Sciences*, *40*(2), 72–78.

Cortassa, S., Caceres, V., Bell, L. N., O'Rourke, B., Paolocci, N., & Aon, M. A. (2015). From metabolomics to fluxomics: A computational procedure to translate metabolite profiles into metabolic fluxes. *Biophysical Journal*, *108*(1), 163–172.

Crittenden, A. N., & Schnorr, S. L. (2017). Current views on hunter-gatherer nutrition and the evolution of the human diet. *American Journal of Physical Anthropology*, *162*, 84–109.

Cyr, A. R., & Domann, F. E. (2011). The redox basis of epigenetic modifications: From mechanisms to functional consequences. *Antioxidants & Redox Signaling*, *15*(2), 551–589.

Dheilly, N. M. (2014). Holobiont–holobiont interactions: Redefining host–parasite interactions. *PLoS Pathogens*, *10*(7), e1004093.

Duncan, E. J., Gluckman, P. D., & Dearden, P. K. (2014). Epigenetics, plasticity, and evolution: How do we link epigenetic change to phenotype? *Journal of Experimental Zoology Part B: Molecular and Developmental Evolution*, *322*(4), 208–220.

Egan, M., Loscri, V., Duong, T. Q., & Di Renzo, M. (2019). Strategies for coexistence in molecular communication. *IEEE Transactions on Nanobioscience*, *18*(1), 51–60.

Ehrenreich, I. M., & Pfennig, D. W. (2015). Genetic assimilation: A review of its potential proximate causes and evolutionary consequences. *Annals of Botany*, *117*(5), 769–779.

Etchegaray, J. P., & Mostoslavsky, R. (2016). Interplay between metabolism and epigenetics: A nuclear adaptation to environmental changes. *Molecular Cell*, *62*(5), 695–711.

Fan, J., Krautkramer, K. A., Feldman, J. L., & Denu, J. M. (2015). Metabolic regulation of histone post-translational modifications. *ACS Chemical Biology*, *10*(1), 95–108.

Fatica, A., & Bozzoni, I. (2014). Long non-coding RNAs: New players in cell differentiation and development. *Nature Reviews Genetics*, *15*(1), 7.

Fondi, M., & Liò, P. (2015). Multi-omics and metabolic modelling pipelines: Challenges and tools for systems microbiology. *Microbiological Research*, *171*, 52–64.

Forman, H. J., Fukuto, J. M., & Torres, M. (2004). Redox signaling: Thiol chemistry defines which reactive oxygen and nitrogen species can act as second messengers. *American Journal of Physiology-Cell Physiology*, *287*(2), C246–C256.

Fox, R. J., Donelson, J. M., Schunter, C., Ravasi, T., & Gaitán-Espitia, J. D. (2019). Beyond buying time: The role of plasticity in phenotypic adaptation to rapid environmental change. *Philosophical Transactions of the Royal Society B: Biological Sciences*, *374*(1768).

Frías-Lasserre, D., & Villagra, C. A. (2017). The importance of ncRNAs as epigenetic mechanisms in phenotypic variation and organic evolution. *Frontiers in Microbiology*, *8*, 2483.

Gluckman, P. D., Low, F. M., Buklijas, T., Hanson, M. A., & Beedle, A. S. (2011). How evolutionary principles improve the understanding of human health and disease. *Evolutionary Applications*, *4*(2), 249–263.

Greer, R., Dong, X., Morgun, A., & Shulzhenko, N. (2016). Investigating a holobiont: Microbiota perturbations and transkingdom networks. *Gut Microbes*, *7*(2), 126–135.

Gutzat, R., & Scheid, O. M. (2012). Epigenetic responses to stress: Triple defense? *Current Opinion in Plant Biology*, *15*(5), 568–573.

Hanly, D. J., Esteller, M., & Berdasco, M. (2018). Interplay between long non-coding RNAs and epigenetic machinery: Emerging targets in cancer? *Philosophical Transactions of the Royal Society B: Biological Sciences*, *373*(1748), 20170074.

He, F., Fromion, V., & Westerhoff, H. V. (2013). (Im) perfect robustness and adaptation of metabolic networks subject to metabolic and gene-expression regulation: Marrying control engineering with metabolic control analysis. *BMC Systems Biology*, *7*(1), 131.

Heard, E., & Martienssen, R. A. (2014). Transgenerational epigenetic inheritance: Myths and mechanisms. *Cell, 157*(1), 95–109.
Holland, M. L. (2017). Epigenetic regulation of the protein translation machinery. *eBioMedicine, 17*, 3–4.
Huang, B., & Zhang, R. (2014). Regulatory non-coding RNAs: Revolutionizing the RNA world. *Molecular Biology Reports, 41*(6), 3915–3923.
Hurst, G. D. (2017). Extended genomes: Symbiosis and evolution. *Interface Focus*, 7(5), 20170001.
Hussa, E. A., & Goodrich-Blair, H. (2013). It takes a village: Ecological and fitness impacts of multipartite mutualism. *Annual Review of Microbiology, 67*, 161–178.
Jandura, A., & Krause, H. M. (2017). The new RNA world: Growing evidence for long non-coding RNA functionality. *Trends in Genetics, 33*(10), 665–676.
Kanherkar, R. R., Bhatia-Dey, N., & Csoka, A. B. (2014). Epigenetics across the human lifespan. *Frontiers in cell and developmental biology, 2*, 49.
King, J. R., Edgar, S., Qiao, K., & Stephanopoulos, G. (2016). Accessing nature's diversity through metabolic engineering and synthetic biology. *F1000Research, 5*, .
Könnyű, B., & Czárán, T. (2011). The evolution of enzyme specificity in the metabolic replicator model of prebiotic evolution. *PLoS One, 6*(6), e20931.
Kriel, A., Bittner, A. N., Kim, S. H., Liu, K., Tehranchi, A. K., Zou, W. Y., … Wang, J. D. (2012). Direct regulation of GTP homeostasis by (p) ppGpp: A critical component of viability and stress resistance. *Molecular Cell, 48*(2), 231–241.
Kun, Á., Szilágyi, A., Könnyű, B., Boza, G., Zachar, I., & Szathmáry, E. (2015). The dynamics of the RNA world: Insights and challenges. *Annals of the New York Academy of Sciences, 1341*(1), 75–95.
Kuo, T. C. Y., Chen, C. H., Chen, S. H., Lu, I. H., Chu, M. J., Huang, L. C., … Chen, L. F. O. (2015). The effect of red light and far-red light conditions on secondary metabolism in agarwood. *BMC Plant Biology, 15*(1), 139.
Kutschera, U. (2018). Systems biology of eukaryotic superorganisms and the holobiont concept. *Theory in Biosciences, 137*(2), 117–131.
Ladurner, A. G. (2006). Rheostat control of gene expression by metabolites. *Molecular Cell, 24*(1), 1–11.
Law, C., Cheung, P., & Adhvaryu, K. (2015). Chemical "diversity" of chromatin through histone variants and histone modifications. *Current Molecular Biology Reports, 1*(1), 39–59.
Lelandais-Brière, C., Sorin, C., Declerck, M., Benslimane, A., Crespi, M., & Hartmann, C. (2010). Small RNA diversity in plants and its impact in development. *Current Genomics, 11*(1), 14–23.
Liu, X., Yang, S., Zhao, M., Luo, M., Yu, C. W., Chen, C. Y., … Wu, K. (2014). Transcriptional repression by histone deacetylases in plants. *Molecular Plant*, 7(5), 764–772.
Lyon, P. (2017). Environmental complexity, adaptability and bacterial cognition: Godfrey-Smith's hypothesis under the microscope. *Biology and Philosophy, 32*(3), 443–465.
Marijuán, P. C., Navarro, J., & del Moral, R. (2015). How the living is in the world: An inquiry into the informational choreographies of life. *Progress in Biophysics and Molecular Biology, 119*(3), 469–480.
Marijuán, P. C., Navarro, J., & del Moral, R. (2018). How prokaryotes 'encode' their environment: Systemic tools for organizing the information flow. *Biosystems, 164*, 26–38.
Markowiak, P., & Śliżewska, K. (2018). The role of probiotics, prebiotics and synbiotics in animal nutrition. *Gut pathogens, 10*(1), 21.
Matzke, M. A., Kanno, T., & Matzke, A. J. (2015). RNA-directed DNA methylation: The evolution of a complex epigenetic pathway in flowering plants. *Annual Review of Plant Biology, 66*, 243–267.
Mazzio, E. A., & Soliman, K. F. (2012). Basic concepts of epigenetics: Impact of environmental signals on gene expression. *Epigenetics*, 7(2), 119–130.

Mazzio, E. A., & Soliman, K. F. (2014). Epigenetics and nutritional environmental signals. *Integrative and Comparative Biology*, *54*(1), 21.
Meier, J. L. (2013). Metabolic mechanisms of epigenetic regulation. *ACS Chemical Biology*, *8*(12), 2607–2621.
Mellin, J. R., & Cossart, P. (2015). Unexpected versatility in bacterial riboswitches. *Trends in Genetics*, *31*(3), 150–156.
Metallo, C. M., & Vander Heiden, M. G. (2013). Understanding metabolic regulation and its influence on cell physiology. *Molecular Cell*, *49*(3), 388–398.
Meyer, P. (2015). Epigenetic variation and environmental change. *Journal of Experimental Botany*, *66*(12), 3541–3548.
Mhlongo, M. I., Piater, L. A., Madala, N. E., Labuschagne, N., & Dubery, I. A. (2018). The chemistry of plant–microbe interactions in the rhizosphere and the potential for metabolomics to reveal signaling related to defense priming and induced systemic resistance. *Frontiers in Plant Science*, *9*, 112.
Miousse, I. R., Currie, R., Datta, K., Ellinger-Ziegelbauer, H., French, J. E., Harrill, A. H., … Moggs, J. G. (2015). Importance of investigating epigenetic alterations for industry and regulators: An appraisal of current efforts by the Health and Environmental Sciences Institute. *Toxicology*, *335*, 11–19.
Mohanty, B. K., & Kushner, S. R. (2018). Enzymes involved in post-transcriptional RNA metabolism in gram-negative bacteria. *Microbiology spectrum*, *6*(2).
Moler, E. R., Abakir, A., Eleftheriou, M., Johnson, J. S., Krutovsky, K. V., Lewis, L. C., … Rajora, O. P. (2018). Population epigenomics: Advancing understanding of phenotypic plasticity, acclimation, adaptation and diseases. In O. P. Rajora (Ed.), *Population genomics* (pp. 179–260). Cham: Springer.
Monaco, P., Marcel, V., Diaz, J. J., & Catez, F. (2018). 2′-O-Methylation of ribosomal RNA: Towards an epitranscriptomic control of translation? *Biomolecules*, *8*(4), 106.
Müller, M. M. (2017). Post-translational modifications of protein backbones: Unique functions, mechanisms, and challenges. *Biochemistry*, *57*(2), 177–185.
Mushegian, A. A., & Ebert, D. (2016). Rethinking "mutualism" in diverse host-symbiont communities. *BioEssays*, *38*(1), 100–108.
Naviaux, R. K. (2018). Metabolic features and regulation of the healing cycle—A new model for chronic disease pathogenesis and treatment. *Mitochondrion*, *46*, 278–297.
Nelson, J. W., Sudarsan, N., Furukawa, K., Weinberg, Z., Wang, J. X., & Breaker, R. R. (2013). Riboswitches in eubacteria sense the second messenger c-di-AMP. *Nature Chemical Biology*, *9*(12), 834.
Nieborak, A., & Schneider, R. (2018). Metabolic intermediates—Cellular messengers talking to chromatin modifiers. *Molecular metabolism*, *14*, 39–52.
Nijhout, H. F., Sadre-Marandi, F., Best, J., & Reed, M. C. (2017). Systems biology of phenotypic robustness and plasticity. *Integrative and Comparative Biology*, *57*(2), 171–184.
Noda-Garcia, L., Liebermeister, W., & Tawfik, D. S. (2018). Metabolite–enzyme coevolution: From single enzymes to metabolic pathways and networks. *Annual Review of Biochemistry*, *87*, 187–216.
Noller, H. F. (2012). Evolution of protein synthesis from an RNA world. *Cold Spring Harbor Perspectives in Biology*, *4*(4), a003681.
Norouzitallab, P., Baruah, K., Vanrompay, D., & Bossier, P. (2018). Can epigenetics translate environmental cues into phenotypes? *The Science of the Total Environment*, *647*, 1281.
Paniagua Voirol, L. R., Frago, E., Kaltenpoth, M., Hilker, M., & Fatouros, N. E. (2018). Bacterial symbionts in lepidoptera: Their diversity, transmission, and impact on the host. *Frontiers in Microbiology*, *9*, 556.
Pfannenstiel, B. T., & Keller, N. P. (2019). On top of biosynthetic gene clusters: How epigenetic machinery influences secondary metabolism in fungi. *Biotechnology Advances*, *37*(6), 107345.

Picard, M., McEwen, B. S., Epel, E. S., & Sandi, C. (2018). An energetic view of stress: Focus on mitochondria. *Frontiers in Neuroendocrinology*, *49*, 72–85.

Pradeu, T. (2016). Organisms or biological individuals? Combining physiological and evolutionary individuality. *Biology and Philosophy*, *31*(6), 797–817.

Qadri, M., Nalli, Y., Jain, S. K., Chaubey, A., Ali, A., Strobel, G. A., … Riyaz-Ul-Hassan, S. (2017). An insight into the secondary metabolism of *Muscodor yucatanensis*: Small-molecule epigenetic modifiers induce expression of secondary metabolism-related genes and production of new metabolites in the endophyte. *Microbial Ecology*, *73*(4), 954–965.

Ramirez-Prado, J. S., Piquerez, S. J., Bendahmane, A., Hirt, H., Raynaud, C., & Benhamed, M. (2018). Modify the histone to win the battle: Chromatin dynamics in plant–pathogen interactions. *Frontiers in Plant Science*, *9*, 355.

Rana, A. K., & Ankri, S. (2016). Reviving the RNA world: An insight into the appearance of RNA methyltransferases. *Frontiers in Genetics*, *7*, 99.

Reen, F., Romano, S., Dobson, A., & O'Gara, F. (2015). The sound of silence: Activating silent biosynthetic gene clusters in marine microorganisms. *Marine Drugs*, *13*(8), 4754–4783.

Reigstad, C. S., & Kashyap, P. C. (2013). Beyond phylotyping: Understanding the impact of gut microbiota on host biology. *Neurogastroenterology & Motility*, *25*(5), 358–372.

Renoz, F., Champagne, A., Degand, H., Faber, A. M., Morsomme, P., Foray, V., & Hance, T. (2017). Toward a better understanding of the mechanisms of symbiosis: A comprehensive proteome map of a nascent insect symbiont. *PeerJ*, *5*, e3291.

Rothbart, S. B., & Strahl, B. D. (2014). Interpreting the language of histone and DNA modifications. *Biochimica et Biophysica Acta (BBA)-Gene Regulatory Mechanisms*, *1839*(8), 627–643.

Roundtree, I. A., Evans, M. E., Pan, T., & He, C. (2017). Dynamic RNA modifications in gene expression regulation. *Cell*, *169*(7), 1187–1200.

Rowland, I., Gibson, G., Heinken, A., Scott, K., Swann, J., Thiele, I., & Tuohy, K. (2018). Gut microbiota functions: Metabolism of nutrients and other food components. *European Journal of Nutrition*, *57*(1), 1–24.

Runcie, A. C., Chan, K. H., Zengerle, M., & Ciulli, A. (2016). Chemical genetics approaches for selective intervention in epigenetics. *Current Opinion in Chemical Biology*, *33*, 186–194.

Ryall, B., Eydallin, G., & Ferenci, T. (2012). Culture history and population heterogeneity as determinants of bacterial adaptation: The adaptomics of a single environmental transition. *Microbiology and Molecular Biology Reviews*, *76*(3), 597–625.

Sandoval-Motta, S., Aldana, M., & Frank, A. (2017). Evolving ecosystems: Inheritance and selection in the light of the microbiome. *Archives of Medical Research*, *48*(8), 780–789.

Santos, R. B., Pires, A. S., & Abranches, R. (2017). Addition of a histone deacetylase inhibitor increases recombinant protein expression in Medicago truncatula cell cultures. *Scientific Reports*, 7(1), 16756.

Schaefer, M., Kapoor, U., & Jantsch, M. F. (2017). Understanding RNA modifications: The promises and technological bottlenecks of the 'epitranscriptome'. *Open Biology*, 7(5), 170077.

Schenk, S. T., Hernández-Reyes, C., Samans, B., Stein, E., Neumann, C., Schikora, M., … Schikora, A. (2014). N-acyl-homoserine lactone primes plants for cell wall reinforcement and induces resistance to bacterial pathogens via the salicylic acid/oxylipin pathway. *The Plant Cell*, *26*(6), 2708–2723.

Schuster, M., Joseph Sexton, D., Diggle, S. P., & Peter Greenberg, E. (2013). Acyl-homoserine lactone quorum sensing: From evolution to application. *Annual Review of Microbiology*, *67*, 43–63.

Schvartzman, J. M., Thompson, C. B., & Finley, L. W. (2018). Metabolic regulation of chromatin modifications and gene expression. *The Journal of Cell Biology*, *217*(7), 2247–2259.

Sergiev, P.V., Aleksashin, N. A., Chugunova, A. A., Polikanov, Y. S., & Dontsova, O. A. (2018). Structural and evolutionary insights into ribosomal RNA methylation. *Nature Chemical Biology*, *14*(3), 226.

Sewelam, N., Kazan, K., & Schenk, P. M. (2016). Global plant stress signaling: Reactive oxygen species at the cross-road. *Frontiers in Plant Science*, 7, 187.

Shalayel, I., Coulibaly, S., Ly, K., Milet, A., & Vallée, Y. (2018). The reaction of aminonitriles with aminothiols: A way to thiol-containing peptides and nitrogen heterocycles in the primitive Earth Ocean. *Life*, *8*(4), 47.

Shapiro, J. (2017). Living organisms author their read-write genomes in evolution. *Biology*, *6*(4), 42.

Shapiro, J. A. (2019). No genome is an island: Toward a 21st century agenda for evolution. *Annals of the New York Academy of Sciences*, *1447*(1), 21–52.

Shen, Y., Torchia, M. L. G., Lawson, G. W., Karp, C. L., Ashwell, J. D., & Mazmanian, S. K. (2012). Outer membrane vesicles of a human commensal mediate immune regulation and disease protection. *Cell Host & Microbe*, *12*(4), 509–520.

Sneppen, K. (2017). Models of life: Epigenetics, diversity and cycles. *Reports on Progress in Physics*, *80*(4), 042601.

Son, J. M., & Lee, C. (2019). Mitochondria: Multifaceted regulators of aging. *BMB Reports*, *52*(1), 13.

Song, J., & Yi, C. (2017). Chemical modifications to RNA: A new layer of gene expression regulation. *ACS Chemical Biology*, *12*(2), 316–325.

Sorek, M., Schnytzer, Y., Ben-Asher, H. W., Caspi, V. C., Chen, C. S., Miller, D. J., & Levy, O. (2018). Setting the pace: Host rhythmic behaviour and gene expression patterns in the facultatively symbiotic cnidarian Aiptasia are determined largely by *Symbiodinium*. *Microbiome*, *6*(1), 83.

Speijer, D. (2017). Alternating terminal electron-acceptors at the basis of symbiogenesis: How oxygen ignited eukaryotic evolution. *BioEssays*, *39*(2), 1600174.

Steinchen, W., & Bange, G. (2016). The magic dance of the alarmones (p) ppGpp. *Molecular Microbiology*, *101*(4), 531–544.

Strauss, J., & Reyes-Dominguez, Y. (2011). Regulation of secondary metabolism by chromatin structure and epigenetic codes. *Fungal Genetics and Biology*, *48*(1), 62–69.

Tammen, S. A., Friso, S., & Choi, S. W. (2013). Epigenetics: The link between nature and nurture. *Molecular Aspects of Medicine*, *34*(4), 753–764.

Thiebaut, F., Hemerly, A. S., & Ferreira, P. C. G. (2019). A role for epigenetic regulation in the adaptation and stress responses of non-model plants. *Frontiers in Plant Science*, *10*, 246.

Thomas, J. M., Batista, P. J., & Meier, J. L. (2019). Metabolic regulation of the epitranscriptome. *ACS Chemical Biology*, *14*(3), 316–324.

Thomas, S., Izard, J., Walsh, E., Batich, K., Chongsathidkiet, P., Clarke, G., … Gilligan, J. P. (2017). The host microbiome regulates and maintains human health: A primer and perspective for non-microbiologists. *Cancer Research*, 77(8), 1783–1812.

Thomas, G. H., Zucker, J., Macdonald, S. J., Sorokin, A., Goryanin, I., & Douglas, A. E. (2009). A fragile metabolic network adapted for cooperation in the symbiotic bacterium *Buchnera aphidicola*. *BMC Systems Biology*, *3*(1), 24.

Torday, J., & Miller, W. (2016). The unicellular state as a point source in a quantum biological system. *Biology*, *5*(2), 25.

Torday, J. S., Miller, W. B., Jr. (2016). Biologic relativity: Who is the observer and what is observed? *Progress in Biophysics and Molecular Biology*, *121*(1), 29–34.

Vallee, Y., Shalayel, I., Ly, K. D., Rao, K. R., De Paëpe, G., Märker, K., & Milet, A. (2017). At the very beginning of life on earth: The thiol-rich peptide (TRP) world hypothesis. *International Journal of Developmental Biology*, *61*(8–9), 471–478.

van de Water, J. A., Allemand, D., & Ferrier-Pagès, C. (2018). Host-microbe interactions in octocoral holobionts-recent advances and perspectives. *Microbiome*, *6*(1), 64.

Vorholt, J. A., Vogel, C., Carlström, C. I., & Mueller, D. B. (2017). Establishing causality: Opportunities of synthetic communities for plant microbiome research. *Cell Host & Microbe*, *22*(2), 142–155.

Wagner, A. (2012). The role of robustness in phenotypic adaptation and innovation. *Proceedings of the Royal Society B: Biological Sciences*, *279*(1732), 1249–1258.

Wang, Y., Liu, H., & Sun, Z. (2017). Lamarck rises from his grave: Parental environment-induced epigenetic inheritance in model organisms and humans. *Biological Reviews*, *92*(4), 2084–2111.

Westerhoff, H. V., Brooks, A. N., Simeonidis, E., García-Contreras, R., He, F., Boogerd, F. C., ... Kolodkin, A. (2014). Macromolecular networks and intelligence in microorganisms. *Frontiers in Microbiology*, *5*, 379.

Xie, P., Zang, L. Q., Li, X. K., & Shu, Q. (2016). An epigenetic view of developmental diseases: New targets, new therapies. *World Journal of Pediatrics*, *12*(3), 291–297.

Yaish, M. W. (2013). *DNA methylation-associated epigenetic changes in stress tolerance of plants*. In *Molecular stress physiology of plants*. India: Springer. (pp. 427–440).

Yaish, M. W. (2017). Epigenetic modifications associated with abiotic and biotic stresses in plants: An implication for understanding plant evolution. *Frontiers in Plant Science*, *8*, 1983.

Yang, T., Owen, J. L., Lightfoot, Y. L., Kladde, M. P., & Mohamadzadeh, M. (2013). Microbiota impact on the epigenetic regulation of colorectal cancer. *Trends in Molecular Medicine*, *19*(12), 714–725.

Zarins-Tutt, J. S., Barberi, T. T., Gao, H., Mearns-Spragg, A., Zhang, L., Newman, D. J., & Goss, R. J. M. (2016). Prospecting for new bacterial metabolites: A glossary of approaches for inducing, activating and upregulating the biosynthesis of bacterial cryptic or silent natural products. *Natural Product Reports*, *33*(1), 54–72.

CHAPTER 7

Systems biology, drug development, and clinical outcomes

We grow in direct proportion to the amount of chaos we can sustain and dissipate

The understanding of complexity and the use of the creativity of nature, the continuation of the work of nature are the grand challenges for the scientists of the 21st century.

Only when a system behaves in a sufficiently random way may the difference between past and future, and therefore irreversibility, enter into its description…The arrow of time is the manifestation of the fact that the future is not given, that, as the French poet Paul Valery emphasized, 'time is a construction.'

Ilya Prigogine (1917–2003)

7.1 Introduction

The biology of systems as a multidisciplinary approach capable of correlating the variables and interactions involved in the evolution and conformation of biological systems is a promising tool for the development of pharmaceutical innovations capable of giving homeostatic equilibrium to the holobiont (Bizzarri, Palombo, & Cucina, 2013; Bowes & Jaffee, 2013). In this way, systems biology can provide models with a high capacity to predict the functioning of drugs and their possible adverse reactions based on their interactions with fitness and adaptation mechanisms (Ayers & Day, 2015; Somvanshi & Venkatesh, 2014). Thus, modeling in systems of metabolic networks, as well as their dynamic modeling, are important tools for translating the knowledge of biomedicine to the discovery of therapeutic innovations (Schleidgen et al., 2017; Schmidt, Papin, & Musante, 2013). Likewise, models of phenotypic adaptations

Molecular Evolutionary Models in Drug Discovery
https://doi.org/10.1016/B978-0-12-817613-9.00007-9

to stress in the pathophysiology of the disease will have a high impact in predicting the behavior of the disruptions of the biological systems that lead to the development of systemic alterations, as well as to determine the targets of therapeutic action that lead to the restoration of balance in the system (Boyce & Ellis, 2005; Heindel et al., 2017). Likewise, determining the mechanisms of epigenetic modifications in response to environmental changes in each holobiont will provide crucial information to predict the clinical outcome of treatment in affected patients (Kramer & Bressan, 2015; Renz et al., 2017).

Equally, the search for drugs capable of maintaining the thermodynamic equilibrium of a living organism, by allowing the sharing of energy from the open system to the environment, is an evolutionary approach that will provide a new framework for pharmacology (Haddad, 2017; Xie et al., 2014). To understand this aspect, it is necessary to correlate the genetic, epigenetic, and environmental factors that modify the action of the drugs in order to understand how the evolutionary adaptations of the individual are a key part of the establishment of a personalized treatment (Baye, Abebe, & Wilke, 2011; Toraño, García, Fernández-Morera, Niño-García, & Fernández, 2016). In this correlation of interacting factors, it is necessary to use computational tools capable of integrating the omics data of the biological system to offer an interactome with which to make applications and choose therapeutic options; this interactome should offer the clinician the evolutionary characteristics of the patient in order to seek the establishment of an organic homeostasis (De Souza, Fiocchi, & Iliopoulos, 2017; Hecker, Lambeck, Toepfer, Van Someren, & Guthke, 2009; Sorger et al., 2011).

In this way, ideas the evolutionary factors of the human patient must include the mechanisms of phenotypic adaptation involved, as well as the description of the symbionts that make up its microbiome and finally the metabolomics of the symbiotic interactions present in the biological system, in order to obtain the individual evolutoma that allows the development of a personalized medicine protocol (Murall et al., 2017; Zaneveld, McMinds, & Thurber, 2017). For this reason, the objective of this chapter is to integrate the mechanisms of adaptation and acquisition of fitness in a systems biology model for the development of a novel approach in the discovery of new drugs and development of new therapies, as well as protocol design of treatment.

7.2 Systems biology in the exposome

The human holobiont is constantly exposed to general and specific external environmental factors, as well as to internal ones in the framework of the interactions it performs; all this exchange, in conjunction with the adaptive response of the biological system, constitutes the exposome (Miller Jr., 2018; Soen, Knafo, & Elgart, 2015). The study of the exposome integrates the adaptive phenotypic capacities of the biological system in response to environmental changes; this response encompasses epigenetic variations as well as the production of bioactive molecules through metabolic networks (Cortese-Krott et al., 2017; Vrijheid, 2014). Although the exposome has been considered as a disease factor, it is necessary to remember that the environmental stress in an evolutionary driver; so the disease can be considered a failure of the biological system in the attempt to reach the homeostatic balance (Dennis & Jones, 2016; Münzel et al., 2016). Thus, the epigenetic responses to the exposome can be classified according to the following criteria (Osamor, Chinedu, Azuh, Iweala, & Ogunlana, 2016; Roundtree & He, 2016):

- pretranscriptional modifications in response to general and specific environmental factors;
- posttranscriptional modifications in response to general and specific environmental factors;
- posttranslational modifications in response to general and specific environmental factors; and
- modifications of biosynthetic pathways in response to molecular signals transduced by the microbiota into the interior of the holobiont.

These epigenetic and epitranscriptomic responses, as well as the balance that the biological system acquires as they are performed, will determine the functionality of the phenotypic adaptations that are carried out since, by not acquiring determined functionality, the fitness will not be possible and the system will fail (Dinescu et al., 2019; Lobo, Barros-Silva, Henrique, & Jerónimo, 2018). In this way, the study of the exposome will give us, in an integral way, the set of environmental factors with which the holobiont interacts, as well as the type of adaptive response that is being developed in order to determine the effective therapeutic approach that will help to restore the balance in the system (Destoumieux-Garzón et al., 2018; Stingone et al., 2017; van Tongeren & Cherrie, 2012).

7.3 Evolutoma and interactomes: Toward a protocol of personalized medicine

In order to establish a protocol of personalized medicine, it is necessary to know the evolutionary capacities of the biological system; this is in order to know the metabolic networks that configure the search for nutrients and competition for space, which is in order to restore its thermodynamic equilibrium (Flores,

Glusman, Brogaard, Price, & Hood, 2013; Houle, Govindaraju, & Omholt, 2010). So in this way, the "4Ps" medicine criterion (predictive, preventive, participatory, and personalized) should include an evolutionary factor that we will call the "fifth P" (pliability) (Auffray, Charron, & Hood, 2010; Sobradillo, Pozo, & Agustí, 2011; Trovato, Catalano, Musumeci, & Trovato, 2014), defining pliability as the adaptive capacity of the biological system in front of the external and internal environmental factors and the evolutionary chemical response that confers plasticity to the holobiont for its transformation and acquisition of fitness (DeBiasse & Kelly, 2015; Reuter, Camus, Hill, Ruzicka, & Fowler, 2017). This is how the biology of systems applied to medicine requires inclusion of evolutionary models for the development of new medicines, procedures, and treatment protocols (Harvey, Edrada-Ebel, & Quinn, 2015; Nowak-Sliwinska et al., 2016). In this way, the integration of adaptome, epigenome, genome, microbiome, metabolome, and exposome becomes necessary in an evolutoma that determines all the characteristics of interaction and symbiosis in the biological system, allowing prediction of the behavior and the clinical outcome (Kopac & Klassen, 2016; Raina et al., 2018). Equally, the disease should be taken as part of the interaction of the holobiont with its environment—all the factors involved in the production and resolution of it are part of a diseaseasome that identifies the disease as an integral process (Chen, Deng, et al., 2018; Chen, Garmaeva, Zhernakova, Fu, & Wijmenga, 2018; DiSalvo, Hatzopolous, & Sawyer, 2015). Finally, by applying coevolution to the health disease duality, the phenomics integration in personalized medicine is the basis for the development of effective diagnostic methods and treatments that can decrease morbidity rates and increase life expectancy.

7.4 Phenomics of personalized medicine

Understanding the phenotypic adaptations that occur in the disease is a principle approach to human evolution (Fay, 2013; Ho & Zhang, 2018; Radwan & Babik, 2012). Thus, in this acquisition of fitness during human evolution, the expression and silencing of several genes that determine the functionality of the biological system have been modulated (Houri-Zeevi & Rechavi, 2017; Ulitsky, 2016). So the disease suffers a phenomenon of adaptation based on the triad of plasticity-relaxation-mutation (PRM) (Hughes, 2012; Snell-Rood, 2012). Among the adaptive phenomena that take place during the disease process are replication, inflammation, and tissue repair (Amor et al., 2014; Chen, Deng, et al., 2018; Chen, Garmaeva, et al., 2018). In this way, a protocol of personalized medicine must determine the biomarkers that determine the phenomics of the inflammatory and repair process in each individual with a view to examining the possible mutation rate that the biological system can present (Giuliani, Garagnani, & Franceschi, 2018; Pasipoularides, 2018). Likewise, the analysis of the inflammatory phenotypes through the phenomic profiles can guide the therapy and the discovery of new drugs that regulate the network of metabolic fluxes that is compromised in the patient (Gu, Crosier, Hall, Chen, & Xu, 2016; Mattick, 2013).

We could say that a more proinflammatory life predisposes to a greater degree of adaptive stress and that the level of inflammation suffered by the holobiont predicts the degree of suffering of the system (Dhabhar, 2014; Grissom, George, & Reyes, 2017). Equally, the homeostasis of the holobiont is a correct balance between the protective factors of inflammation and the mutational consequences of chronicity (Chovatiya & Medzhitov, 2014; Wiesner & Klein, 2017). On the other hand, we should analyze the role that epigenetics has in the adaptive inflammatory response, where the regulation of the expression of TNF-α (tumor necrosis factor), interleukins, tumor suppressor genes, oncogenes, and the transcription factor NF-kB are the targets of the modifications (Jones et al., 2016; Shanmugam & Sethi, 2013). This means that the adaptive processes that lead to the biological diversity of the biological system for its survival are relapsing on the proinflammatory factors and that these induce the production of secondary metabolites that, in turn, induce further modifications that lead to the change of the hologenome (O'Malley & Skillings, 2018; Selber-Hnatiw et al., 2017). So that's where we begin to discern that a personalized medicine analyzes the disruption of symbiosis during the adaptation phenomenon, that is, the dysbiosis that chronifies the disease and produces mutagenesis (Huang et al., 2017; Livnat, 2017); thus, the pliability within the 5Ps studies and correlates the individual variations within the symbiotic relationships that keep the holobiont in balance and that allow its survival in the face of adaptation (Eloe-Fadrosh & Rasko, 2013; Gilbert et al., 2010).

7.5 Systems biology and symbiosis in homeostasis

The mutualistic interactions between the symbionts and the host make up the equilibrium of the holobiont; its disruption is the dysbiosis, and it alters the homeostasis and the state of health of the biological system by inducing chronic inflammatory phenomena (Carrier & Reitzel, 2017; Kutschera, 2018). The phenomics of dysbiosis is an unregulated response to the production of secondary metabolites (e.g., butyrate, propionate, acetate, succinate, deoxycholate, and lithocholate), as well as the expression of biosynthetic enzymes that prolong the nonequilibrium state that predisposes to the appearance of non-adaptive mutations in the hologenome, which affects their organization (Chen & Stappenbeck, 2019; Hall et al., 2018; Miller, Svanbäck, & Bohannan, 2018). This is how the pharmacological search of homeostasis for the treatment of patients should be oriented toward the design of therapies that maintain the symbiosis within the holobiont; that is, toward the design of symbiotic medications (Kuntz & Gilbert, 2017; Mao & Franke, 2015). In this way, symbiotic medication must seek to restore the homeostasis of the biological system; this is achieved by regulating the adaptive processes to environmental changes within the holobiont, avoiding the chronicity of the conditions and dysbiosis (Garcia & Gerardo, 2014; Haque & Haque, 2017). Likewise, restoring the functional population of symbionts in interaction with the host is a trait that should be considered by personalized medicine, because it can alter the pharmacokinetics and pharmacodynamics of the therapy (Armstrong, Lee, & Armstrong, 2018; Gurwitz, 2013; Ramos, Callier, & Rotimi, 2012).

So in this way, the microbiota can biotransform the drugs, as well as alter their absorption and distribution, which would lead to therapeutic failure (Choi, Yu, Yoo, & Kim, 2018; Enright, Gahan, Joyce, & Griffin, 2016; Wilkinson, Ilhan, & Herbst-Kralovetz, 2018). In addition, the microbiome establishes functional symbiosis when it is in a state of equilibrium; on the other hand, the dysbiosis increases the inflammation and with this, reduces the absorption and biodistribution of the drugs (Ballal, Gallini, Segata, Huttenhower, & Garrett, 2011; Moya & Ferrer, 2016). Likewise, the use of strategies for the design of new drugs that preserve homeostasis in the holobiont must use symbiotic approaches where the complementary biological functions with which to develop hybrid drugs are directed to both the healing and maintenance of the functional populations of interacting symbionts with the host (Kothari, Koringa, & Singh, 2017; Pommier & Cherfils, 2005). Thus, knowledge of the patient's hologenome becomes a priority to determine the functional populations of the symbionts involved and to try to predict the adaptive responses of the host, and to solve this type of question, the use of metagenomics is required (Foster, Schluter, Coyte, & Rakoff-Nahoum, 2017; Knight et al., 2012; Stencel & Wloch-Salamon, 2018).

7.6 Metagenomics in personalized medicine and drug development: The microbiome makes the holobiont

Metagenomics is a promising tool capable of identifying the populations of organisms within the holobiont, as well as the enzymes and metabolites involved in symbiosis (Karimi et al., 2017; Suenaga, 2015). This discipline applied in environmental ecology has the ability to reveal the interaction characteristics of individual ecosystems from the analysis of the total genetic material of environmental samples, and will have a great impact on personalized medicine if the patient is examined as an eco-evolutionary entity (Ezard, Côté, & Pelletier, 2009; Palkovacs & Hendry, 2010; Penczykowski, Laine, & Koskella, 2016). So, as an eco-evolutionary entity has a development based on the interactions between the environment, its symbionts, and the host, this determines its predisposition and resistance to the disease as a disruptive phenomenon (Dheilly, Poulin, & Thomas, 2015; Koskella, Hall, & Metcalf, 2017; Macke, Tasiemski, Massol, Callens, & Decaestecker, 2017). In this way, high-performance sequencing, in conjunction with computer tools, can offer us an overview of the community metabolism, as well as the metabolic networks established for each ecosystem individual (Kreimer, Doron-Faigenboim, Borenstein, & Freilich, 2012; Logares et al., 2012; Mahadevan & Henson, 2012).

In addition, the correlation of the community metabolism with the genotypic identification of the species in mutualist interaction will allow us to know the behavior of the hologenome as a whole against environmental challenges, as well as the direct response of the holobiont to the exposome (Freilich et al., 2011; McClure et al., 2018). Likewise, in determining the degree of interspecies exchange that occurs in each individual, metagenomic diagnosis can promote personalized medicine based on the patient's functionality as an ecosystem (Robinson, Bohannan, & Young, 2010; Virgin & Todd, 2011). Equally, the value of metagenomics is the ability to provide global information about the biological system, both of the symbiotic populations involved and of the genomic alterations caused by dysbiosis, which offers a new platform for evaluating the biological activity of medicines where it can know both the degree of involvement and monitor the recovery of the patient with the therapy administered (Contreras, Cocom-Chan, Hernandez-Montes, Portillo-Bobadilla, & Resendis-Antonio, 2016; Morgan & Huttenhower, 2012; Wang & Jia, 2016). Thus, metagenomics will be a fundamental piece in the monitoring of novel approaches for the evaluation of the activity, the effectiveness, and the adverse reactions of symbiotic drugs with which to reestablish the metabolic networks and the symbiosis in the human biological system (Louca & Doebeli, 2015; Woyke et al., 2006).

7.7 Symbiotic approaches in the development of new drugs, balance, pliability, adaptation, and healing

The symbiotic approach to the development of medicines seeks to obtain hybrid molecules with different biological activities in order to carry out a multitarget therapy (Cardona-G, Yepes, & Herrera-R, 2018; Decker, 2011; Simone Tranches Dias & Viegas, 2014). This multitarget therapy should be focused on the four principles of personalized medicine, but it is important to add the implications for the phenotypic adaptations of the host that the design of these drugs may affect (Martin, Phillips, Thomas, & Somogyi, 2015; Mathur & Sutton, 2017; Verweij, de Jonge, Eskens, & Sleijfer, 2012). It is also important to determine for each new medication the epigenetic modifications that this can induce and the type of change that these compounds can cause on the methylation of DNA and RNA, as well as in the acetylation or deacetylation of histones (Heerboth et al., 2014; Kelly, De Carvalho, & Jones, 2010; Reuter, Gupta, Park, Goel, & Aggarwal, 2011). Likewise, the use of epigenetic modifications as a target for the action of drugs in order to regulate adaptive responses to the exposome may be an important therapeutic strategy to avoid mutations resulting from chronic diseases (Carroll et al., 2014; Coyle, Boudreau, & Marcato, 2017). Additionally, the restoration of functional populations of symbionts should be a priority issue for the development of new drugs, either to treat the disruption of symbiosis produced by dysbiosis, or to improve the absorption and bioavailability of medications (Ercolini & Fogliano, 2018; Holmes et al., 2012; Picca et al., 2018). Thus, the biology of systems allows the patient to assume as an eco-evolutionary individual that has to be in balance with their environment to which they are constantly adapting; so a global vision of drug discovery is necessary that does not evaluate the specialized therapeutic target in isolation, but also determines the interaction and communication signals that pharmacological intervention can cause (Koparde, Doijad, & Magdum, 2019; Thomford et al., 2018).

7.8 Conclusions

A therapeutic approach that assumes the patient as a holobiont in constant evolution in interaction and adaptation with their environment will be key to the development of novel diagnostic techniques as well as the discovery of new drugs (Bueno, 2017; Miller Jr., 2016). It will also be possible to predict the clinical outcome based on the behavior of the symbioses, the functional populations that make up the biological system as well as the reestablishment of the metabolic networks that regulate energy pathways in an open system such as the human body (Dominguez-Bello, Godoy-Vitorino, Knight, & Blaser, 2019; Hadrich, 2018). Likewise, the challenge is to study the individual as an eco-evolutionary system that acquires the disease by disruption of its molecular communication becoming chronic, and the lack of regulation of the phenotypic adaptations that underlie it (Hendry, 2015; Loeuille, 2019). So, this perspective does not develop a personalized medicine under the criterion of precision, but it is possible to conceive medicine as an evolutionary system of a biology that makes each adaptive process unique within an ecosystem (Bircher & Hahn, 2016; Ching et al., 2018). Finally, the cure is achieved under the treatment resulting from the deep understanding of the disease as a phenomenon linked to the evolution of the human being as a biological system belonging to a particular biosphere, not as an isolated entity, but as a unit of a metaholobiont (van de Guchte, Blottière, & Doré, 2018).

References

Amor, S., Peferoen, L. A., Vogel, D. Y., Breur, M., van der Valk, P., Baker, D., & van Noort, J. M. (2014). Inflammation in neurodegenerative diseases—An update. *Immunology*, *142*(2), 151–166.

Armstrong, L. E., Lee, E. C., & Armstrong, E. M. (2018). Interactions of gut microbiota, endotoxemia, immune function, and diet in exertional heatstroke. *The Journal of Sports Medicine*, *2018*, 5724575.

Auffray, C., Charron, D., & Hood, L. (2010). Predictive, preventive, personalized and participatory medicine: Back to the future. *Genome Medicine*, *2*(8), 57.

Ayers, D., & Day, P. J. (2015). Systems medicine: The application of systems biology approaches for modern medical research and drug development. *Molecular Biology International*, *2015*, 698169.

Ballal, S. A., Gallini, C. A., Segata, N., Huttenhower, C., & Garrett, W. S. (2011). Host and gut microbiota symbiotic factors: Lessons from inflammatory bowel disease and successful symbionts. *Cellular Microbiology*, *13*(4), 508–517.

Baye, T. M., Abebe, T., & Wilke, R. A. (2011). Genotype–environment interactions and their translational implications. *Personalized Medicine*, *8*(1), 59–70.

Bircher, J., & Hahn, E. G. (2016). Applying a complex adaptive system's understanding of health to primary care. *F1000Research*, *5*.

Bizzarri, M., Palombo, A., & Cucina, A. (2013). Theoretical aspects of systems biology. *Progress in Biophysics and Molecular Biology*, *112*(1–2), 33–43.

Bowes, L., & Jaffee, S. R. (2013). Biology, genes, and resilience: Toward a multidisciplinary approach. *Trauma, Violence & Abuse*, *14*(3), 195–208.

Boyce, W. T., & Ellis, B. J. (2005). Biological sensitivity to context: I. An evolutionary–developmental theory of the origins and functions of stress reactivity. *Development and Psychopathology*, *17*(2), 271–301.

Bueno, J. (2017). The future of metabolomics and individual monitoring in antimicrobial therapy. *Journal of Microbial & Biochemical Technology*, *9*, e132.

Cardona-G, W., Yepes, A. F., & Herrera-R, A. (2018). Hybrid molecules: Promising compounds for the development of new treatments against Leishmaniasis and Chagas disease. *Current Medicinal Chemistry*, *25*(30), 3637–3679.

Carrier, T. J., & Reitzel, A. M. (2017). The hologenome across environments and the implications of a host-associated microbial repertoire. *Frontiers in Microbiology, 8*, 802.

Carroll, S. P., Jørgensen, P. S., Kinnison, M. T., Bergstrom, C. T., Denison, R. F., Gluckman, P., … Tabashnik, B. E. (2014). Applying evolutionary biology to address global challenges. *Science, 346*(6207), 1245993.

Chen, L., Deng, H., Cui, H., Fang, J., Zuo, Z., Deng, J., … Zhao, L. (2018). Inflammatory responses and inflammation-associated diseases in organs. *Oncotarget, 9*(6), 7204.

Chen, L., Garmaeva, S., Zhernakova, A., Fu, J., & Wijmenga, C. (2018). A system biology perspective on environment–host–microbe interactions. *Human Molecular Genetics, 27*(R2), R187–R194.

Chen, F., & Stappenbeck, T. S. (2019). Microbiome control of innate reactivity. *Current Opinion in Immunology, 56*, 107–113.

Ching, T., Himmelstein, D. S., Beaulieu-Jones, B. K., Kalinin, A. A., Do, B. T., Way, G. P., … Xie, W. (2018). Opportunities and obstacles for deep learning in biology and medicine. *Journal of the Royal Society Interface, 15*(141), 20170387.

Choi, M. S., Yu, J. S., Yoo, H. H., & Kim, D. H. (2018). The role of gut microbiota in the pharmacokinetics of antihypertensive drugs. *Pharmacological Research, 130*, 164–171.

Chovatiya, R., & Medzhitov, R. (2014). Stress, inflammation, and defense of homeostasis. *Molecular Cell, 54*(2), 281–288.

Contreras, A.V., Cocom-Chan, B., Hernandez-Montes, G., Portillo-Bobadilla, T., & Resendis-Antonio, O. (2016). Host-microbiome interaction and cancer: Potential application in precision medicine. *Frontiers in Physiology, 7*, 606.

Cortese-Krott, M. M., Koning, A., Kuhnle, G. G., Nagy, P., Bianco, C. L., Pasch, A., … Olson, K. R. (2017). The reactive species interactome: Evolutionary emergence, biological significance, and opportunities for redox metabolomics and personalized medicine. *Antioxidants & Redox Signaling, 27*(10), 684–712.

Coyle, K. M., Boudreau, J. E., & Marcato, P. (2017). Genetic mutations and epigenetic modifications: Driving cancer and informing precision medicine. *BioMed Research International, 2017*.

De Souza, H. S., Fiocchi, C., & Iliopoulos, D. (2017). The IBD interactome: An integrated view of aetiology, pathogenesis and therapy. *Nature Reviews Gastroenterology & Hepatology, 14*(12), 739.

DeBiasse, M. B., & Kelly, M. W. (2015). Plastic and evolved responses to global change: What can we learn from comparative transcriptomics? *Journal of Heredity, 107*(1), 71–81.

Decker, M. (2011). Hybrid molecules incorporating natural products: Applications in cancer therapy, neurodegenerative disorders and beyond. *Current Medicinal Chemistry, 18*(10), 1464–1475.

Dennis, K. K., & Jones, D. P. (2016). The exposome: A new frontier for education. *The American Biology Teacher, 78*(7), 542–548.

Destoumieux-Garzón, D., Mavingui, P., Boetsch, G., Boissier, J., Darriet, F., Duboz, P., … Paillard, C. (2018). The one health concept: 10 years old and a long road ahead. *Frontiers in Veterinary Science, 5*, 14.

Dhabhar, F. S. (2014). Effects of stress on immune function: The good, the bad, and the beautiful. *Immunologic Research, 58*(2–3), 193–210.

Dheilly, N. M., Poulin, R., & Thomas, F. (2015). Biological warfare: Microorganisms as drivers of host–parasite interactions. *Infection, Genetics and Evolution, 34*, 251–259.

Dinescu, S., Ignat, S., Lazar, A. D., Constantin, C., Neagu, M., & Costache, M. (2019). Epitranscriptomic signatures in lncRNAs and their possible roles in cancer. *Genes, 10*(1), 52.

DiSalvo, T. G., Hatzopolous, A., & Sawyer, D. (2015). TGFβ, Wnt/β-catenin and hippo pathway "Cross-talk": Myocardial systems biology murmurings as the pathways converge. *Journal of Advances in Medicine and Medical Research*, 16–47.

Dominguez-Bello, M. G., Godoy-Vitorino, F., Knight, R., & Blaser, M. J. (2019). Role of the microbiome in human development. *Gut*, *68*(6), 1108–1114.
Eloe-Fadrosh, E. A., & Rasko, D. A. (2013). The human microbiome: From symbiosis to pathogenesis. *Annual Review of Medicine*, *64*, 145–163.
Enright, E. F., Gahan, C. G., Joyce, S. A., & Griffin, B. T. (2016). Focus: Microbiome: The impact of the gut microbiota on drug metabolism and clinical outcome. *The Yale Journal of Biology and Medicine*, *89*(3), 375.
Ercolini, D., & Fogliano, V. (2018). Food design to feed the human gut microbiota. *Journal of Agricultural and Food Chemistry*, *66*(15), 3754–3758.
Ezard, T. H., Côté, S. D., & Pelletier, F. (2009). Eco-evolutionary dynamics: Disentangling phenotypic, environmental and population fluctuations. *Philosophical Transactions of the Royal Society, B: Biological Sciences*, *364*(1523), 1491–1498.
Fay, J. C. (2013). Disease consequences of human adaptation. *Applied & Translational Genomics*, *2*, 42–47.
Flores, M., Glusman, G., Brogaard, K., Price, N. D., & Hood, L. (2013). P4 medicine: How systems medicine will transform the healthcare sector and society. *Personalized Medicine*, *10*(6), 565–576.
Foster, K. R., Schluter, J., Coyte, K. Z., & Rakoff-Nahoum, S. (2017). The evolution of the host microbiome as an ecosystem on a leash. *Nature*, *548*(7665), 43.
Freilich, S., Zarecki, R., Eilam, O., Segal, E. S., Henry, C. S., Kupiec, M., … Ruppin, E. (2011). Competitive and cooperative metabolic interactions in bacterial communities. *Nature Communications*, *2*, 589.
Garcia, J. R., & Gerardo, N. M. (2014). The symbiont side of symbiosis: Do microbes really benefit? *Frontiers in Microbiology*, *5*, 510.
Gilbert, S. F., McDonald, E., Boyle, N., Buttino, N., Gyi, L., Mai, M., … Robinson, J. (2010). Symbiosis as a source of selectable epigenetic variation: Taking the heat for the big guy. *Philosophical Transactions of the Royal Society, B: Biological Sciences*, *365*(1540), 671–678.
Giuliani, C., Garagnani, P., & Franceschi, C. (2018). Genetics of human longevity within an eco-evolutionary nature-nurture framework. *Circulation Research*, *123*(7), 745–772.
Grissom, N. M., George, R., & Reyes, T. M. (2017). Suboptimal nutrition in early life affects the inflammatory gene expression profile and behavioral responses to stressors. *Brain, Behavior, and Immunity*, *63*, 115–126.
Gu, J., Crosier, P. S., Hall, C. J., Chen, L., & Xu, X. (2016). Inflammatory pathway network-based drug repositioning and molecular phenomics. *Molecular BioSystems*, *12*(9), 2777–2784.
Gurwitz, D. (2013). The gut microbiome: Insights for personalized medicine. *Drug Development Research*, *74*(6), 341–343.
Haddad, W. (2017). Thermodynamics: The unique universal science. *Entropy*, *19*(11), 621.
Hadrich, D. (2018). Microbiome research is becoming the key to better understanding health and nutrition. *Frontiers in Genetics*, *9*.
Hall, E. K., Bernhardt, E. S., Bier, R. L., Bradford, M. A., Boot, C. M., Cotner, J. B., … Lennon, J. T. (2018). Understanding how microbiomes influence the systems they inhabit. *Nature Microbiology*, *3*(9), 977.
Haque, S. Z., & Haque, M. (2017). The ecological community of commensal, symbiotic, and pathogenic gastrointestinal microorganisms—An appraisal. *Clinical and Experimental Gastroenterology*, *10*, 91.
Harvey, A. L., Edrada-Ebel, R., & Quinn, R. J. (2015). The re-emergence of natural products for drug discovery in the genomics era. *Nature Reviews Drug Discovery*, *14*(2), 111.
Hecker, M., Lambeck, S., Toepfer, S., Van Someren, E., & Guthke, R. (2009). Gene regulatory network inference: Data integration in dynamic models—A review. *Biosystems*, *96*(1), 86–103.

Heerboth, S., Lapinska, K., Snyder, N., Leary, M., Rollinson, S., & Sarkar, S. (2014). Use of epigenetic drugs in disease: An overview. *Genetics & Epigenetics*, *6*, GEG-S12270.
Heindel, J. J., Blumberg, B., Cave, M., Machtinger, R., Mantovani, A., Mendez, M. A., … Vandenberg, L. N. (2017). Metabolism disrupting chemicals and metabolic disorders. *Reproductive Toxicology*, *68*, 3–33.
Hendry, A. P. (2015). Key questions on the role of phenotypic plasticity in eco-evolutionary dynamics. *Journal of Heredity*, *107*(1), 25–41.
Ho, W. C., & Zhang, J. (2018). Evolutionary adaptations to new environments generally reverse plastic phenotypic changes. *Nature Communications*, *9*(1), 350.
Holmes, E., Kinross, J., Gibson, G. R., Burcelin, R., Jia, W., Pettersson, S., & Nicholson, J. K. (2012). Therapeutic modulation of microbiota-host metabolic interactions. *Science Translational Medicine*, *4*(137), 137rv6.
Houle, D., Govindaraju, D. R., & Omholt, S. (2010). Phenomics: The next challenge. *Nature Reviews Genetics*, *11*(12), 855.
Houri-Zeevi, L., & Rechavi, O. (2017). A matter of time: Small RNAs regulate the duration of epigenetic inheritance. *Trends in Genetics*, *33*(1), 46–57.
Huang, Y. J., Marsland, B. J., Bunyavanich, S., O'Mahony, L., Leung, D. Y., Muraro, A., & Fleisher, T. A. (2017). The microbiome in allergic disease: Current understanding and future opportunities—2017 PRACTALL document of the American Academy of Allergy, Asthma & Immunology and the European Academy of Allergy and Clinical Immunology. *Journal of Allergy and Clinical Immunology*, *139*(4), 1099–1110.
Hughes, A. L. (2012). Evolution of adaptive phenotypic traits without positive Darwinian selection. *Heredity*, *108*(4), 347.
Jones, V. S., Huang, R. Y., Chen, L. P., Chen, Z. S., Fu, L., & Huang, R. P. (2016). Cytokines in cancer drug resistance: Cues to new therapeutic strategies. *Biochimica et Biophysica Acta*, *1865*(2), 255–265.
Karimi, E., Ramos, M., Gonçalves, J., Xavier, J. R., Reis, M. P., & Costa, R. (2017). Comparative metagenomics reveals the distinctive adaptive features of the *Spongia officinalis* endosymbiotic consortium. *Frontiers in Microbiology*, *8*, 2499.
Kelly, T. K., De Carvalho, D. D., & Jones, P. A. (2010). Epigenetic modifications as therapeutic targets. *Nature Biotechnology*, *28*(10), 1069.
Knight, R., Jansson, J., Field, D., Fierer, N., Desai, N., Fuhrman, J. A., … Bailey, M. J. (2012). Unlocking the potential of metagenomics through replicated experimental design. *Nature Biotechnology*, *30*(6), 513.
Kopac, S. M., & Klassen, J. L. (2016). Can they make it on their own? Hosts, microbes, and the holobiont niche. *Frontiers in Microbiology*, 7, 1647.
Koparde, A. A., Doijad, R. C., & Magdum, C. S. (2019). Natural products in drug discovery. In S. Perveen & A. Al-Taweel (Eds.), *Pharmacognosy—Medicinal plants*. London: IntechOpen.
Koskella, B., Hall, L. J., & Metcalf, C. J. E. (2017). The microbiome beyond the horizon of ecological and evolutionary theory. *Nature Ecology & Evolution*, *1*(11), 1606.
Kothari, R., Koringa, P. G., & Singh, S. P. (2017). In R. P. Singh (Ed.), *Understanding host-microbiome Interactions: An omics approach*. Cham: Springer.
Kramer, P., & Bressan, P. (2015). Humans as superorganisms: How microbes, viruses, imprinted genes, and other selfish entities shape our behavior. *Perspectives on Psychological Science*, *10*(4), 464–481.
Kreimer, A., Doron-Faigenboim, A., Borenstein, E., & Freilich, S. (2012). NetCmpt: A network-based tool for calculating the metabolic competition between bacterial species. *Bioinformatics*, *28*(16), 2195–2197.
Kuntz, T. M., & Gilbert, J. A. (2017). Introducing the microbiome into precision medicine. *Trends in Pharmacological Sciences*, *38*(1), 81–91.
Kutschera, U. (2018). Systems biology of eukaryotic superorganisms and the holobiont concept. *Theory in Biosciences*, *137*(2), 117–131.

Livnat, A. (2017). Simplification, innateness, and the absorption of meaning from context: How novelty arises from gradual network evolution. *Evolutionary Biology*, *44*(2), 145–189.

Lobo, J., Barros-Silva, D., Henrique, R., & Jerónimo, C. (2018). The emerging role of epitranscriptomics in cancer: Focus on urological tumors. *Genes*, *9*(11), 552.

Loeuille, N. (2019). Eco-evolutionary dynamics in a disturbed world: Implications for the maintenance of ecological networks. *F1000Research*, *8*.

Logares, R., Haverkamp, T. H., Kumar, S., Lanzén, A., Nederbragt, A. J., Quince, C., & Kauserud, H. (2012). Environmental microbiology through the lens of high-throughput DNA sequencing: Synopsis of current platforms and bioinformatics approaches. *Journal of Microbiological Methods*, *91*(1), 106–113.

Louca, S., & Doebeli, M. (2015). Calibration and analysis of genome-based models for microbial ecology. *eLife*, *4*, e08208.

Macke, E., Tasiemski, A., Massol, F., Callens, M., & Decaestecker, E. (2017). Life history and eco-evolutionary dynamics in light of the gut microbiota. *Oikos*, *126*(4), 508–531.

Mahadevan, R., & Henson, M. A. (2012). Genome-based modeling and design of metabolic interactions in microbial communities. *Computational and Structural Biotechnology Journal*, *3*(4), e201210008.

Mao, L., & Franke, J. (2015). Symbiosis, dysbiosis, and rebiosis—The value of metaproteomics in human microbiome monitoring. *Proteomics*, *15*(5–6), 1142–1151.

Martin, J. H., Phillips, E., Thomas, D., & Somogyi, A. A. (2015). Adding the 'medicines' back into personalized medicine to improve cancer treatment outcomes. *British Journal of Clinical Pharmacology*, *80*(5), 929–931.

Mathur, S., & Sutton, J. (2017). Personalized medicine could transform healthcare. *Biomedical Reports*, 7(1), 3–5.

Mattick, J. S. (2013). Genetics: Probing the phenomics of noncoding RNA. *eLife*, *2*, e01968.

McClure, R. S., Overall, C. C., Hill, E. A., Song, H. S., Charania, M., Bernstein, H. C., … Beliaev, A. S. (2018). Species-specific transcriptomic network inference of interspecies interactions. *The ISME Journal*, *12*(8), 2011.

Miller, W. B., Jr. (2016). The eukaryotic microbiome: Origins and implications for fetal and neonatal life. *Frontiers in Pediatrics*, *4*, 96.

Miller, W. B., Jr. (2018). Biological information systems: Evolution as cognition-based information management. *Progress in Biophysics and Molecular Biology*, *134*, 1–26.

Miller, E. T., Svanbäck, R., & Bohannan, B. J. M. (2018). Microbiomes as metacommunities: Understanding host-associated microbes through metacommunity ecology. *Trends in Ecology & Evolution*, *33*(12), 926–935.

Morgan, X. C., & Huttenhower, C. (2012). Human microbiome analysis. *PLoS Computational Biology*, *8*(12), e1002808.

Moya, A., & Ferrer, M. (2016). Functional redundancy-induced stability of gut microbiota subjected to disturbance. *Trends in Microbiology*, *24*(5), 402–413.

Münzel, T., Sørensen, M., Gori, T., Schmidt, F. P., Rao, X., Brook, F. R., … Rajagopalan, S. (2016). Environmental stressors and cardio-metabolic disease: Part II–mechanistic insights. *European Heart Journal*, *38*(8), 557–564.

Murall, C. L., Abbate, J. L., Touzel, M. P., Allen-Vercoe, E., Alizon, S., Froissart, R., & McCann, K. (2017). *Invasions of host-associated microbiome networks*. In Vol. 57. *Advances in ecological research*. Academic Press. (pp. 201–281).

Nowak-Sliwinska, P., Weiss, A., Ding, X., Dyson, P. J., Van Den Bergh, H., Griffioen, A. W., & Ho, C. M. (2016). Optimization of drug combinations using feedback system control. *Nature Protocols*, *11*(2), 302.

O'Malley, M. A., & Skillings, D. J. (2018). Methodological strategies in microbiome research and their explanatory implications. *Perspectives on Science*, *26*(2), 239–265.

Osamor, V. C., Chinedu, S. N., Azuh, D. E., Iweala, E. J., & Ogunlana, O. O. (2016). The interplay of post-translational modification and gene therapy. *Drug Design, Development and Therapy, 10*, 861.
Palkovacs, E. P., & Hendry, A. P. (2010). Eco-evolutionary dynamics: Intertwining ecological and evolutionary processes in contemporary time. *F1000 Biology Reports, 2*.
Pasipoularides, A. (2018). Implementing genome-driven personalized cardiology in clinical practice. *Journal of Molecular and Cellular Cardiology, 115*, 142–157.
Penczykowski, R. M., Laine, A. L., & Koskella, B. (2016). Understanding the ecology and evolution of host–parasite interactions across scales. *Evolutionary Applications, 9*(1), 37–52.
Picca, A., Fanelli, F., Calvani, R., Mulè, G., Pesce, V., Sisto, A., … Marzetti, E. (2018). Gut dysbiosis and muscle aging: Searching for novel targets against sarcopenia. *Mediators of Inflammation, 2018*, 7026198.
Pommier, Y., & Cherfils, J. (2005). Interfacial inhibition of macromolecular interactions: Nature's paradigm for drug discovery. *Trends in Pharmacological Sciences, 26*(3), 138–145.
Radwan, J., & Babik, W. (2012). The genomics of adaptation. *Proceedings of the Royal Society B: Biological Sciences, 279*(1749), 5024.
Raina, J. B., Eme, L., Pollock, F. J., Spang, A., Archibald, J. M., & Williams, T. A. (2018). Symbiosis in the microbial world: From ecology to genome evolution. *Biology Open, 7*(2), bio032524.
Ramos, E., Callier, S. L., & Rotimi, C. N. (2012). Why personalized medicine will fail if we stay the course. *Personalized Medicine, 9*(8), 839–847.
Renz, H., Holt, P. G., Inouye, M., Logan, A. C., Prescott, S. L., & Sly, P. D. (2017). An exposome perspective: Early-life events and immune development in a changing world. *Journal of Allergy and Clinical Immunology, 140*(1), 24–40.
Reuter, M., Camus, M. F., Hill, M. S., Ruzicka, F., & Fowler, K. (2017). Evolving plastic responses to external and genetic environments. *Trends in Genetics, 33*(3), 169–170.
Reuter, S., Gupta, S. C., Park, B., Goel, A., & Aggarwal, B. B. (2011). Epigenetic changes induced by curcumin and other natural compounds. *Genes & Nutrition, 6*(2), 93.
Robinson, C. J., Bohannan, B. J., & Young, V. B. (2010). From structure to function: The ecology of host-associated microbial communities. *Microbiology and Molecular Biology Reviews, 74*(3), 453–476.
Roundtree, I. A., & He, C. (2016). RNA epigenetics—Chemical messages for posttranscriptional gene regulation. *Current Opinion in Chemical Biology, 30*, 46–51.
Schleidgen, S., Fernau, S., Fleischer, H., Schickhardt, C., Oßa, A. K., & Winkler, E. C. (2017). Applying systems biology to biomedical research and health care: A précising definition of systems medicine. *BMC Health Services Research, 17*(1), 761.
Schmidt, B. J., Papin, J. A., & Musante, C. J. (2013). Mechanistic systems modeling to guide drug discovery and development. *Drug Discovery Today, 18*(3–4), 116–127.
Selber-Hnatiw, S., Rukundo, B., Ahmadi, M., Akoubi, H., Al-Bizri, H., Aliu, A. F., … Begum, F. (2017). Human gut microbiota: Toward an ecology of disease. *Frontiers in Microbiology, 8*, 1265.
Shanmugam, M. K., & Sethi, G. (2013). *Role of epigenetics in inflammation-associated diseases*. In *Epigenetics: Development and disease*. Dordrecht: Springer. (pp. 627–657).
Simone Tranches Dias, K., & Viegas, C. (2014). Multi-target directed drugs: A modern approach for design of new drugs for the treatment of Alzheimer's disease. *Current Neuropharmacology, 12*(3), 239–255.
Snell-Rood, E. C. (2012). Selective processes in development: Implications for the costs and benefits of phenotypic plasticity. *Integrative and Comparative Biology, 52*(1), 31.
Sobradillo, P., Pozo, F., & Agustí, Á. (2011). P4 medicine: The future around the corner. *Archivos de Bronconeumología, 47*(1), 35–40.
Soen, Y., Knafo, M., & Elgart, M. (2015). A principle of organization which facilitates broad Lamarckian-like adaptations by improvisation. *Biology Direct, 10*(1), 68.

Somvanshi, P. R., & Venkatesh, K.V. (2014). A conceptual review on systems biology in health and diseases: From biological networks to modern therapeutics. *Systems and Synthetic Biology*, *8*(1), 99–116.

Sorger, P. K., Allerheiligen, S. R., Abernethy, D. R., Altman, R. B., Brouwer, K. L., Califano, A., ... Lauffenburger, D. A. (2011, October). *Quantitative and systems pharmacology in the post-genomic era: New approaches to discovering drugs and understanding therapeutic mechanisms.* In: *an nih white paper by the QSP workshop group*.Vol. 48. Bethesda, MD: NIH.

Stencel, A., & Wloch-Salamon, D. M. (2018). Some theoretical insights into the hologenome theory of evolution and the role of microbes in speciation. *Theory in Biosciences*, *137*(2), 197–206.

Stingone, J. A., Buck Louis, G. M., Nakayama, S. F., Vermeulen, R. C., Kwok, R. K., Cui, Y., ... Teitelbaum, S. L. (2017). Toward greater implementation of the exposome research paradigm within environmental epidemiology. *Annual Review of Public Health*, *38*, 315–327.

Suenaga, H. (2015). Targeted metagenomics unveils the molecular basis for adaptive evolution of enzymes to their environment. *Frontiers in Microbiology*, *6*, 1018.

Thomford, N., Senthebane, D., Rowe, A., Munro, D., Seele, P., Maroyi, A., & Dzobo, K. (2018). Natural products for drug discovery in the 21st century: Innovations for novel drug discovery. *International Journal of Molecular Sciences*, *19*(6), 1578.

Toraño, E. G., García, M. G., Fernández-Morera, J. L., Niño-García, P., & Fernández, A. F. (2016). The impact of external factors on the epigenome: In utero and over lifetime. *BioMed Research International*, *2016*.

Trovato, F. M., Catalano, D., Musumeci, G., & Trovato, G. M. (2014). 4Ps medicine of the fatty liver: The research model of predictive, preventive, personalized and participatory medicine—Recommendations for facing obesity, fatty liver and fibrosis epidemics. *The EPMA Journal*, *5*(1), 21.

Ulitsky, I. (2016). Evolution to the rescue: Using comparative genomics to understand long non-coding RNAs. *Nature Reviews Genetics*, *17*(10), 601.

van de Guchte, M., Blottière, H. M., & Doré, J. (2018). Humans as holobionts: Implications for prevention and therapy. *Microbiome*, *6*(1), 81.

van Tongeren, M., & Cherrie, J. W. (2012). An integrated approach to the exposome. *Environmental Health Perspectives*, *120*(3), a103–a104.

Verweij, J., de Jonge, M., Eskens, F., & Sleijfer, S. (2012). Moving molecular targeted drug therapy towards personalized medicine: Issues related to clinical trial design. *Molecular Oncology*, *6*(2), 196–203.

Virgin, H. W., & Todd, J. A. (2011). Metagenomics and personalized medicine. *Cell*, *147*(1), 44–56.

Vrijheid, M. (2014). The exposome: A new paradigm to study the impact of environment on health. *Thorax*, *69*(9), 876–878.

Wang, J., & Jia, H. (2016). Metagenome-wide association studies: Fine-mining the microbiome. *Nature Reviews Microbiology*, *14*(8), 508.

Wiesner, D. L., & Klein, B. S. (2017). The balance between immunity and inflammation. *Science*, *357*(6355), 973–974.

Wilkinson, E. M., Ilhan, Z. E., & Herbst-Kralovetz, M. M. (2018). Microbiota–drug interactions: Impact on metabolism and efficacy of therapeutics. *Maturitas*, *112*, 53–63.

Woyke, T., Teeling, H., Ivanova, N. N., Huntemann, M., Richter, M., Gloeckner, F. O., ... Szeto, E. (2006). Symbiosis insights through metagenomic analysis of a microbial consortium. *Nature*, *443*(7114), 950.

Xie, L., Ge, X., Tan, H., Xie, L., Zhang, Y., Hart, T., ... Bourne, P. E. (2014). Towards structural systems pharmacology to study complex diseases and personalized medicine. *PLoS Computational Biology*, *10*(5), e1003554.

Zaneveld, J. R., McMinds, R., & Thurber, R.V. (2017). Stress and stability: Applying the Anna Karenina principle to animal microbiomes. *Nature Microbiology*, *2*(9), 17121.

CHAPTER 8

Toxical autopoiesis

In a sense it has been my way to transcendental experience: to the discovery that matter metaphorically speaking, is the creation of the spirit (the mode of existence of the observer in a domain of discourse), and that the spirit is the creation of the matter it creates. This is not a paradox, but it is the expression of our existence in a domain of cognition in which the content of cognition is cognition itself. Beyond that nothing can be said.

Living systems are units of interactions; they exist in an ambience. From a purely biological point of view they cannot be understood independently of that part of the ambience with which they interact: the niche; nor can the niche be defined independently of the living system that specifies it.

Man knows and his capacity to know depends on his biological integrity; furthermore, he knows that he knows. As a basic psychological and, hence, biological function cognition guides his handling of the universe and knowledge gives certainty to his acts; objective knowledge seems possible and through objective knowledge the universe appears systematic and predictable.

Humberto Maturana (1928–)

8.1 Introduction

By definition, an autopoietic system is one that reproduces itself; that is, acquires replicative capacity by being able to adapt to its environment and enter into equilibrium (Baum, 2018; Lane, 2018; Razeto-Barry, 2012). Thus, a biological system becomes autopoietic when it develops chemical and physical processes that establish metabolic networks with which to have a flow of obtaining energy (Lomas & Giampietro, 2017; Lucia & Grisolia, 2017; Zivieri, Pacini, Finocchio, & Carpentieri, 2017). Likewise, the processes become autopoietic when they allow phenotypic adaptation mediated epigenetically with respect to environmental changes; that is, they allow cognition and learning of the environment that surrounds the

Molecular Evolutionary Models in Drug Discovery
https://doi.org/10.1016/B978-0-12-817613-9.00008-0

biological system (Braun, 2015; Stotz & Allen, 2012; Wallace & Wallace, 2009). So an important evolutionary factor is the adaptive learning of what represents a toxic and harmful agent for the biological system, as well as the epigenetic modifications that are carried out by virtue of the damage and the chemical disorder (Calabrese, Cornelius, Dinkova-Kostova, Calabrese, & Mattson, 2010; Charlesworth, Barton, & Charlesworth, 2017; Guthman & Mansfield, 2013). In this way, for a biological system to acquire cognition and self-reference takes its autopoiesis; to achieve this, the cell, the organism, and the holobiont as a whole must know to distinguish between the beneficial and the harmful for the system (Dollens, 2015; Farnsworth, 2018).

Thus the capacity of bioremediation of a system is assumed as much by the interaction as by the structuring of a memory of the information collected to pass to the next generation (Naylor et al., 2017; Zengler, 2009). This means that to acquire the ability to adapt phenotypically and reproduce in an hostile environment, one must have chemical sensors that recognize and stimulate the organism at low doses of exposure and also inhibit high doses of exposure in an evolutionary hormesis model (Agathokleous, Kitao, & Calabrese, 2018a; Costantini, 2014; Hadacek, Bachmann, Engelmeier, & Chobot, 2011). So adaptation and conditioning occurs in response to low doses of the stress agent, which allows self-replication and self-organization within the system and also induces the formation of a memory for survival (Mansouri, Xie, & Rappolee, 2012; Stockhorst & Antov, 2016; Vargas-Hernandez et al., 2017). This phenomenon especially occurs during the oxidative stress mediated by the reactive oxygen species (ROS), so the sensors of chemical signals are conditioned to perceive and respond to this type of compounds (Di Meo, Reed, Venditti, & Victor, 2016; Dickinson & Chang, 2011; Kurutas, 2015).

It is also important to bear in mind that the response of secondary metabolism within the biological system to a prolonged oxidative response is the production of antioxidant compounds capable of regulating the response to achieve fitness (Borecky & Pamenter, 2017; Kasote, Katyare, Hegde, & Bae, 2015; Niinemets et al., 2017). In addition, these antioxidant compounds have the evolutionary role of optimizing the metabolic networks that use oxygen in the production of energy from the nutrients, thus obtaining the functionality of both nutrition and defense (Racchi, 2013; Rahal et al., 2014; Tripathy & Oelmüller, 2012). For the above reasons, the objective of this chapter is to analyze the stimulatory and inhibitory responses to stressors and how they play a fundamental role in the acquisition of autopoiesis, self-reference, and cognition within biological systems, as well as the application of these concepts in the pliability of personalized medicine for the development of innovations in health, agriculture and industry (Blaschke, 2008).

8.2 Evolutionary hormesis

Hormesis is considered the capacity of biological systems to respond to low exposures of environmental stressors with a stimulation of reproduction and a phenotypic adaptation that leads to tolerance to the challenge (Fig. 1) (Calabrese & Mattson, 2011; Costantini, 2019). This is how the hormetic response to toxic agents is mediated by ROS receptors that are sensitive to the redox signals that come from the system (Calabrese et al., 2012; Holmström & Finkel, 2014; Schieber & Chandel, 2014). Then ROS, when firing the hormesis, induces epigenetic modifications, increase of the transcription of factors of proliferation, and differentiation in the DNA, as well as the production of secondary metabolites with the realization of molecular communication and regulation of the metabolic networks (Jacobo-Velázquez, González-Agüero, & Cisneros-Zevallos, 2015; Leak et al., 2015; Medina et al., 2015). Likewise, the phenomenon of hormesis can be regulated by the antioxidant compounds produced under oxidative stress, which indicates that the response loses intensity over time (Calabrese et al., 2007; Damiani et al., 2018; Ristow & Schmeisser, 2014). Likewise, chronic exposure to stressors overcomes the response of hormesis, inducing mutation due to errors in replication (Kim, Hwang, & Choi, 2018; Kim, Lee, Choi, Jacobs

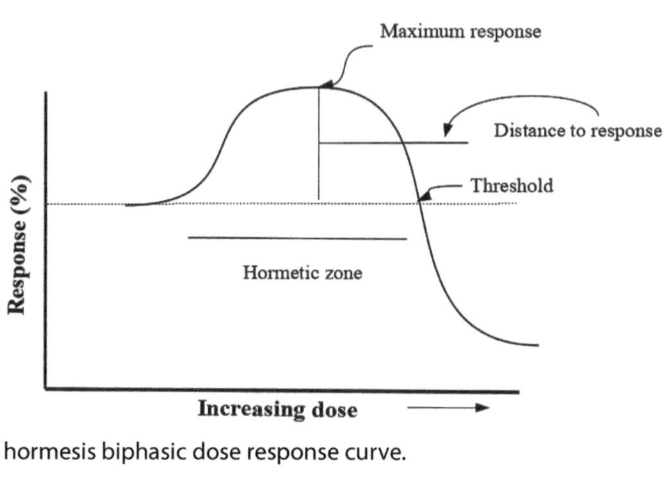

Fig. 1 The hormesis biphasic dose response curve.

Jr., & Lee, 2018; Oh, Lee, & Wagers, 2014; Scott, 2014). Therefore, hormesis is considered as a promoter of evolutionary change, leading to nonlethal mutations that acquire functionality and fitness within the biological system (Calabrese, 2018; Langie et al., 2015; Nei & Nozawa, 2011).

The mitochondria play a fundamental role in this stress response, inducing the production of ROS, inducing nuclear response and tolerance, a phenomenon described as mitohormesis (Fig. 2) (De Haes et al., 2014; Owusu-Ansah, Song, & Perrimon, 2013; Yun & Finkel, 2014). On the other hand, it is important to bear in mind that bacteria also present the phenomenon of hormesis, as demonstrated by resistance due to the indiscriminate use of antibiotics, and thanks to the fact of the endosymbiosis that led to the mitochondria in the eukaryotic cell (Bhakta-Guha & Efferth, 2015; Calabrese, 2014; Weis, 2012). So we can conclude that by producing ROS in response to toxic agents, the microbiome induces proliferation and adaptation within the host; this means that microbial hormesis has been important in the functionality of the microbiota and homeostasis inside the holobiont (Kim, Hwang, et al., 2018; Kim, Lee, et al., 2018; Li et al., 2017; Spooner & Yilmaz, 2011). For this reason, it is important to evaluate the role of hormesis in the response to ROS in the origin of life and how it favors the sharing of entropy to achieve thermodynamic equilibrium in biological systems (Calabrese, Calabrese, & Giordano, 2017; Gatenby & Frieden, 2013; Nunn, Guy, & Bell, 2016, 2017).

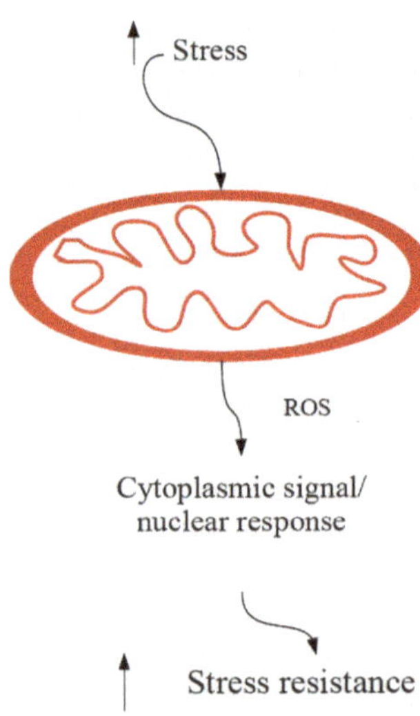

Fig. 2 The basis of mitohormesis.

8.3 ROS in the RNA world

Since the emergence of the proto-cell, which developed a respiratory chain in the cell membrane in order to obtain energy, it became necessary to detect and respond to environmental toxic agents (e.g., ionizing radiation) and induce ROS to activate adaptation phenomena (Azzam, Jay-Gerin, & Pain, 2012; Di Meo et al., 2016; Zorov, Juhaszova, & Sollott, 2014). Thus, the cellular membrane as a biosensor acquired signaling characteristics that allowed it to transduce signals to activate RNA replication, as well as transcription and translation in the riboswitches (Breaker, 2012; Henkin, 2008; Machtel, Bąkowska-Żywicka, & Żywicki, 2016). All this was done in order to protect the RNA, which is very sensitive to oxidative stress, and prevent its degradation due to environmental challenges (Lobo, Patil, Phatak, & Chandra, 2010; Poljsak, 2011; Sharma, Jha, Dubey, & Pessarakli, 2012). Likewise, oxidative stress promoted the evolution of microbial pro-biofilm variants via second messengers, such as cyclic GMP, in order to increase cell resistance and tolerance (Chua et al., 2016; Koo, Allan, Howlin, Stoodley, & Hall-Stoodley, 2017; Römling & Balsalobre, 2012). Thus, it has been shown that the phenomenon of hormesis accelerates the formation of microbial biofilms in response to oxidative stress and light; this tells us of the antiquity of this mechanism of adaptation to acquire fitness capacity (Cui et al., 2018; Kumar et al., 2019; Zheng et al., 2018).

There is also a connection between the fundamental bacterial processes, such as biofilm formation and chemotaxis, and the response to oxidative stress mediated by small RNAs, which suggests that our biology has been used and molded in response to physical and chemical agents with toxicity for biological systems (Čáp, Váchová, & Palková, 2012; Jakubowski & Walkowiak, 2015; Pandin, Le Coq, Canette, Aymerich, & Briandet, 2017). These small noncoding RNAs (sRNAs) are part of the adaptive phenotypic response and the epigenetic regulation of transcription, which integrates evolutionary hormesis with the epigenetic modifications that induce the biosynthesis of new molecules capable of allowing survival and persistence (Blignaut, 2012; Frías-Lasserre & Villagra, 2017; John & Rougeulle, 2018). Thus, the hormesis in the RNA world was a determining factor for the establishment of the adaptive plasticity of the proto cells, as well as the response to oxidative stress to protect the encoded information and the primitive metabolic networks, preparing the way for one of the major innovations in biological systems: the endosymbiosis that led to the appearance of mitochondria (Delaye & Lazcano, 2005; Meléndez-Hevia, Montero-Gómez, & Montero, 2008; Muller, 2005).

8.4 Mitohormesis as an adaptative response

The initial microbial hormesis against stress favored the endosymbiotic coupling that led to mitochondria and mitohormesis was an adaptive innovation (Shadel & Horvath, 2015; Sies, 2019; Son & Lee, 2019). In this way, the phenomenon of mitohormesis allows epigenetic modifications for the adaptation and establishment of metabolic networks in the acquisition of homeostasis via chemical signaling (Etchegaray & Mostoslavsky, 2016; Gabory, Attig, & Junien, 2011; Matilainen, Quirós, & Auwerx, 2017). Thus, mitohormesis in response to oxidative stress induces the pathway of the TOR kinase, which is also sensitive to the presence or absence of nutrients; this path to integrate energy search and chemical defense becomes the signaling path for adaptation (Bitto, Wang, Bennett, & Kaeberlein, 2015; Poljsak, 2011; Swinnen, Ghillebert, Wilms, & Winderickx, 2014). Likewise, the pathway of the TOR kinase is involved in the formation of biofilms by fungi as a means of persistence in the face of environmental challenges (Abdallah, Benoliel, Drider, Dhulster, & Chihib, 2014; Prasad, Shah, & Dhamgaye, 2014; Villa, Cappitelli, Cortesi, & Kunova, 2017). In a similar way, mitohormesis also promotes the response to chemical signals coming from the microbial world, such as quorum sensing molecules, establishing a connection between prokaryotic and eukaryotic cells present both in polymicrobial biofilms and in the interaction between the microbiome and the host (Adhikari, Kwon, Hargis, & Téllez, 2018; Douglas, 2014; Laforest-Lapointe & Arrieta, 2018). Genetic plasticity is another of the evolutionary factors induced by the phenomenon of mitohormesis, which induces change and mutation to achieve the thermodynamic equilibrium of the metabolic pathways (Jones & Robinson, 2018; Leak et al., 2018; Rodriguez, Snoek, Riksen, Bevers, & Kammenga, 2012).

This ROS induction by the mitochondria in response to environmental changes promotes proliferation at low doses, but its persistence over time can lead to failures in adaptation inducing metabolic disorders in the biological system (Liguori et al., 2018; Solleiro-Villavicencio & Rivas-Arancibia, 2018; Tan et al., 2016). Epigenetic modifications of the expression of BGCs lead to the production of chemically diverse antioxidant compounds to regulate prolonged mitochondrial hormesis (Ballard & Youngson, 2015; Gillespie, Pickering, & Eskiw, 2016; Guillaumet-Adkins et al., 2017). Likewise, a superabundance of antioxidant compounds to regulate ROS produced in the phenomenon of mitohormesis can inhibit the adaptive response and prevent adaptation to low doses of exposure (Barbieri et al., 2013; Bárcena, Mayoral,

& Quirós, 2018;Valero, 2014). Thus, the search for homeostasis in hormesis favors the acquisition of fitness in the holobiont, which is where it is part of the mutualistic interaction (Chirumbolo & Bjørklund, 2017; Fratantonio, Cimino, Speciale, & Virgili, 2018; Parashar, Gideon, & Manoj, 2018).

8.5 Microbiomes and the proteasome, endoplasmic reticulum, and mitochondria (PERM) hypothesis

The proteasome, endoplasmic reticulum, and mitochondria (PERM) hypothesis postulates that xenobiotics can modulate oxidative stress in the "proterome" that involves homeostatic mechanisms in the proteasome (P), endoplasmic reticulum (ER), and mitochondria (M) (Bjørklund & Chirumbolo, 2017; Segref et al., 2014; Suliman & Piantadosi, 2016). Inside the holobiont, the symbionts send chemical signals to the host induced by the presence of xenobiotics for active oxidative stress pathways in the biological system (Clarke et al., 2019; El-Demerdash, Tousson, Kurzepa, & Habib, 2018; Postler & Ghosh, 2017). Thus, the PERM hypothesis suggests that the epigenetic response to xenobiotics has been an evolutionary driver of speciation impact (Oliver & Greene, 2011; Slaveykova, Sonntag, & Gutiérrez, 2016;Varriale, 2014). It is also important to take into account the response in the presence of xenobiotic agents by the microbiome, where oxidative stress promotes the exchange of information through the transposable elements (TEs) (Chen & Li, 2007; Mateo, Ullastres, & González, 2014; Miousse et al., 2015). Likewise, TEs influence the modifications of the expression in eukaryotes of the genes that codify for cytochromes P450 that metabolize xenobiotic agents (Kuno, Hirayama-Kurogi, Ito, & Ohtsuki, 2016, 2019;Tizioto et al., 2016).

So in this way, we find that TE-Thrust hypothesis is complementary to the PERM hypothesis, as the oxidative stress and its adaptive response induce the genetic exchange in the hologenome (Lee, Ayarpadikannan, & Kim, 2016; Miller, 2016; Oliver & Greene, 2011). For these reasons, it can be considered that the microbiome functions both as a bioremediation barrier against toxic agents and as a transducer of alert signals and adaptation to the host (Ilangumaran & Smith, 2017; Mhlongo, Piater, Madala, Labuschagne, & Dubery, 2018; Monteverde et al., 2018). So the hormesis in the microbiome is a chemical signal mediated by ROS that induces the genetic exchange in the host to acquire fitness in the form of protective responses (Hansen, Rubinsztein, & Walker, 2018; Miller, Villamena, & Volek, 2018; Naviaux, 2014); that is, the symbionts give information and cognition to the host in the structuring of the holobiont (Limborg & Heeb, 2018; Simon, Marchesi, Mougel, & Selosse, 2019).

8.6 Hormesis, autopoiesis, and drug discovery

In this way, an open biological system that exchanges information as well as energy, and which responds together to external aggressions, has greater adaptive capacities (Picard, McEwen, Epel, & Sandi, 2018; Restivo, 2018). These capabilities allow it to self-replicate against xenobiotic exposure and induced oxidative stress (Jones, Rayson, Flemming, & Urwin, 2013; Siriwardena, 2014). This is how a new approach in the discovery of new drugs is possible, in which the hormetic response is used as a mechanism of action that induces adaptation through epigenetic regulation in the biological system (Vaiserman, 2011). In this order of ideas, by boosting the hormone response both in the microbiome and in the host, ROS production is induced at low exposure doses, which in a controlled manner leads to stimulation in the acquisition of fitness and homeostasis (Belkaid & Hand, 2014; Bhatt, Redinbo, & Bultman, 2017; Wu & Wu, 2012). Likewise, the possibility of pharmacologically modulating the adaptive response of the holobiont using the signaling molecules of hormesis known as hormetins or stressors can induce tolerance, resilience, and increase in the longevity of the biological system (Awasthi, Ramana, Chaudhary, Srivastava, & Awasthi, 2017; Pennisi et al., 2017; Rattan, Sejersen, Fernandes, & Luo, 2007). In this way, hormetins as medicines can be useful to achieve functionality in the balance of biological systems; also these compounds, such as flavonoids, polyphenols, and other algae isolates, act via hormesis and maintain the functional structure by adaptive response to oxidative stress (Rattan, 2012, 2014). Thus, the pharmacological activation of the adaptive response to xenobiotics induces the activation of remediation mechanisms within the holobiont, mechanisms that modify the hologenome and allow resilience and persistence, as well as the permanence of the symbiosis (Haiser & Turnbaugh, 2013; Spanogiannopoulos, Bess, Carmody, & Turnbaugh, 2016).

8.7 Conclusions

A biological system, by becoming autopoietic, becomes self-replicating and acquires adaptive capacity as it interacts with the surrounding environment. In this way, any system should respond to the presence of xenobiotic agents that enter or are present in the ecosystem niche; so in exercising this response, the system acquires the necessary fitness to maintain the mutualistic relationships that allow homeostasis (Di Bernardo, 2010; Segré, Shenhav, Kafri, & Lancet, 2001). Likewise, the symbiosis within the holobiont develops together a hormetic response in order to guarantee the stability of established metabolic networks (Salvioli et al., 2016; Vaiserman, 2010). This response, mediated by ROS, promotes both the chemical signals of proliferative stimulation both in the symbionts and in the host, and is able to induce changes in hologenome by genetic exchange through TEs (Milani et al., 2017; Münger, Montiel-Castro, Langhans, & Pacheco-López, 2018). Likewise, this phenomenon of hormesis causes the holobiont as a whole to acquire cognition of the surrounding environment, in order to adapt in coevolution with other systems of the metaholobiont (Agathokleous, Kitao, & Calabrese, 2018b). Finally, this phenomenon of molecular evolution is the key in the search for new promising compounds known as hormetins, whose mechanism of action is to promote oxidative stress mediated by ROS at low doses of exposure and allow the functioning of the structure of the biological system by inducing its proliferation and exchange of genetic and chemical information, which opens the possibilities to novel therapies that seek the maintenance of homeostasis inside the symbiotic holobiont (Shimi & Goldman, 2014).

References

Abdallah, M., Benoliel, C., Drider, D., Dhulster, P., & Chihib, N. E. (2014). Biofilm formation and persistence on abiotic surfaces in the context of food and medical environments. *Archives of Microbiology, 196*(7), 453–472.

Adhikari, B., Kwon, Y. M., Hargis, B., & Téllez, G. (2018). Prokaryotes rule the world. In A. Evrensel & B.Ö. Ünsalver (Eds.), *Gut microbiota-brain axis* (pp. 2–18). London: IntechOpen.

Agathokleous, E., Kitao, M., & Calabrese, E. J. (2018a). Biphasic effect of abscisic acid on plants: An hormetic viewpoint. *Botany, 96*(10), 637–642.

Agathokleous, E., Kitao, M., & Calabrese, E. J. (2018b). Environmental hormesis and its fundamental biological basis: Rewriting the history of toxicology. *Environmental Research, 165*, 274–278.

Awasthi, Y. C., Ramana, K.V., Chaudhary, P., Srivastava, S. K., & Awasthi, S. (2017). Regulatory roles of glutathione-S-transferases and 4-hydroxynonenal in stress-mediated signaling and toxicity. *Free Radical Biology and Medicine, 111*, 235–243.

Azzam, E. I., Jay-Gerin, J. P., & Pain, D. (2012). Ionizing radiation-induced metabolic oxidative stress and prolonged cell injury. *Cancer Letters, 327*(1–2), 48–60.

Ballard, J. W. O., & Youngson, N. A. (2015). Can diet influence the selective advantage of mitochondrial DNA haplotypes? *Bioscience Reports, 35*(6), e00277.

Barbieri, E., Sestili, P., Vallorani, L., Guescini, M., Calcabrini, C., Gioacchini, A. M., … Stocchi, V. (2013). Mitohormesis in muscle cells: A morphological, molecular, and proteomic approach. *Muscles, Ligaments and Tendons Journal, 3*(4), 254.

Bárcena, C., Mayoral, P., & Quirós, P. M. (2018). Mitohormesis, an antiaging paradigm. *International Review of Cell and Molecular Biology, 340*, 35.

Baum, D. A. (2018). The origin and early evolution of life in chemical composition space. *Journal of Theoretical Biology, 456*, 295–304.

Belkaid, Y., & Hand, T. W. (2014). Role of the microbiota in immunity and inflammation. *Cell, 157*(1), 121–141.

Bhakta-Guha, D., & Efferth, T. (2015). Hormesis: Decoding two sides of the same coin. *Pharmaceuticals, 8*(4), 865–883.

Bhatt, A. P., Redinbo, M. R., & Bultman, S. J. (2017). The role of the microbiome in cancer development and therapy. *CA: A Cancer Journal for Clinicians*, *67*(4), 326–344.
Bitto, A., Wang, A. M., Bennett, C. F., & Kaeberlein, M. (2015). Biochemical genetic pathways that modulate aging in multiple species. *Cold Spring Harbor Perspectives in Medicine*, *5*(11), a025114.
Bjørklund, G., & Chirumbolo, S. (2017). Role of oxidative stress and antioxidants in daily nutrition and human health. *Nutrition*, *33*, 311–321.
Blaschke, S. (2008). *Structures and dynamics of autopoietic organizations: Theory and simulation.* Wiesbaden: Springer Fachmedien Wiesbaden GmbH.
Blignaut, M. (2012). Review of non-coding RNAs and the epigenetic regulation of gene expression: A book edited by Kevin Morris. *Epigenetics*, 7(6), 664–666.
Borecky, L., & Pamenter, M. (2017). Oxygen sensing and transcriptional regulation of adaptive hypoxic responses. In M. Brandt (Ed.), *Chemosensory sensors and systems: Evolutionary significance, biological effects and new insights* (pp. 1–72). NY, USA: Nova Science Publishers.
Braun, C. M. (2015). Biological costs of the evolution of adaptive behavior and consciousness. *Psychology of Consciousness: Theory, Research, and Practice*, *2*(4), 377.
Breaker, R. R. (2012). Riboswitches and the RNA world. *Cold Spring Harbor Perspectives in Biology*, *4*(2), a003566.
Calabrese, E. J. (2014). Hormesis: A fundamental concept in biology. *Microbial Cell*, *1*(5), 145.
Calabrese, E. (2018). Hormesis: Path and progression to significance. *International Journal of Molecular Sciences*, *19*(10), 2871.
Calabrese, E. J., Bachmann, K. A., Bailer, A. J., Bolger, P. M., Borak, J., Cai, L., … Cook, R. R. (2007). Biological stress response terminology: Integrating the concepts of adaptive response and preconditioning stress within a hormetic dose–response framework. *Toxicology and Applied Pharmacology*, *222*(1), 122–128.
Calabrese, E. J., Calabrese, V., & Giordano, J. (2017). The role of hormesis in the functional performance and protection of neural systems. *Brain Circulation*, *3*(1), 1.
Calabrese, V., Cornelius, C., Dinkova-Kostova, A. T., Calabrese, E. J., & Mattson, M. P. (2010). Cellular stress responses, the hormesis paradigm, and vitagenes: Novel targets for therapeutic intervention in neurodegenerative disorders. *Antioxidants & Redox Signaling*, *13*(11), 1763–1811.
Calabrese, V., Cornelius, C., Dinkova-Kostova, A. T., Iavicoli, I., Di Paola, R., Koverech, A., … Calabrese, E. J. (2012). Cellular stress responses, hormetic phytochemicals and vitagenes in aging and longevity. *Biochimica et Biophysica Acta (BBA)-Molecular Basis of Disease*, *1822*(5), 753–783.
Calabrese, E. J., & Mattson, M. P. (2011). Hormesis provides a generalized quantitative estimate of biological plasticity. *Journal of Cell Communication and Signaling*, *5*(1), 25–38.
Čáp, M., Váchová, L., & Palková, Z. (2012). Reactive oxygen species in the signaling and adaptation of multicellular microbial communities. *Oxidative Medicine and Cellular Longevity*, *2012*.
Charlesworth, D., Barton, N. H., & Charlesworth, B. (2017). The sources of adaptive variation. *Proceedings of the Royal Society B: Biological Sciences*, *284*(1855), 20162864.
Chen, S., & Li, X. (2007). Transposable elements are enriched within or in close proximity to xenobiotic-metabolizing cytochrome P450 genes. *BMC Evolutionary Biology*, 7(1), 46.
Chirumbolo, S., & Bjørklund, G. (2017). PERM hypothesis: The fundamental machinery able to elucidate the role of xenobiotics and hormesis in cell survival and homeostasis. *International Journal of Molecular Sciences*, *18*(1), 165.
Chua, S. L., Ding, Y., Liu, Y., Cai, Z., Zhou, J., Swarup, S., … Yang, L. (2016). Reactive oxygen species drive evolution of pro-biofilm variants in pathogens by modulating cyclic-di-GMP levels. *Open Biology*, *6*(11), 160162.
Clarke, G., Sandhu, K. V., Griffin, B. T., Dinan, T. G., Cryan, J. F., & Hyland, N. P. (2019). Gut reactions: Breaking down xenobiotic–microbiome interactions. *Pharmacological Reviews*, *71*(2), 198–224.

Costantini, D. (2014). *Oxidative stress and hormesis in evolutionary ecology and physiology*. Wiesbaden: Springer Fachmedien Wiesbaden GmbH.

Costantini, D. (2019). Hormesis promotes evolutionary change. *Dose-Response*, *17*(2), 1559325819843376.

Cui, X., Huo, M., Chen, C., Yu, Z., Zhou, C., Li, A., … Crittenden, J. C. (2018). Low concentrations of Al (III) accelerate the formation of biofilm: Multiple effects of hormesis and flocculation. *Science of the Total Environment*, *634*, 516–524.

Damiani, E., Brugè, F., Cirilli, I., Marcheggiani, F., Olivieri, F., Armeni, T., … Tiano, L. (2018). Modulation of oxidative status by normoxia and hypoxia on cultures of human dermal fibroblasts: How does it affect cell aging? *Oxidative Medicine and Cellular Longevity*, *2018*.

De Haes, W., Frooninckx, L., Van Assche, R., Smolders, A., Depuydt, G., Billen, J., … Temmerman, L. (2014). Metformin promotes lifespan through mitohormesis via the peroxiredoxin PRDX-2. *Proceedings of the National Academy of Sciences*, *111*(24), E2501–E2509.

Delaye, L., & Lazcano, A. (2005). Prebiological evolution and the physics of the origin of life. *Physics of Life Reviews*, *2*(1), 47–64.

Di Bernardo, M. (2010). Natural selection and self-organization in complex adaptive systems. *Rivista di Biologia*, *103*(1), 89.

Di Meo, S., Reed, T. T., Venditti, P., & Victor, V. M. (2016). Role of ROS and RNS sources in physiological and pathological conditions. *Oxidative Medicine and Cellular Longevity*, *2016*.

Dickinson, B. C., & Chang, C. J. (2011). Chemistry and biology of reactive oxygen species in signaling or stress responses. *Nature Chemical Biology*, 7(8), 504.

Dollens, D. (2015). Autopoiesis+ extended cognition+ nature= can buildings think? *Communicative & Integrative Biology*, *8*(4), e994373.

Douglas, A. E. (2014). Symbiosis as a general principle in eukaryotic evolution. *Cold Spring Harbor Perspectives in Biology*, *6*(2), a016113.

El-Demerdash, F. M., Tousson, E. M., Kurzepa, J., & Habib, S. L. (2018). Xenobiotics, oxidative stress, and antioxidants. *Oxidative Medicine and Cellular Longevity*, *2018*.

Etchegaray, J. P., & Mostoslavsky, R. (2016). Interplay between metabolism and epigenetics: A nuclear adaptation to environmental changes. *Molecular Cell*, *62*(5), 695–711.

Farnsworth, K. (2018). How organisms gained causal independence and how it might be quantified. *Biology*, 7(3), 38.

Fratantonio, D., Cimino, F., Speciale, A., & Virgili, F. (2018). Need (more than) two to tango: Multiple tools to adapt to changes in oxygen availability. *BioFactors*, *44*(3), 207–218.

Frías-Lasserre, D., & Villagra, C. A. (2017). The importance of ncRNAs as epigenetic mechanisms in phenotypic variation and organic evolution. *Frontiers in Microbiology*, *8*, 2483.

Gabory, A., Attig, L., & Junien, C. (2011). Epigenetic mechanisms involved in developmental nutritional programming. *World Journal of Diabetes*, *2*(10), 164.

Gatenby, R. A., & Frieden, B. R. (2013). The critical roles of information and nonequilibrium thermodynamics in evolution of living systems. *Bulletin of Mathematical Biology*, *75*(4), 589–601.

Gillespie, Z. E., Pickering, J., & Eskiw, C. H. (2016). Better living through chemistry: Caloric restriction (CR) and CR mimetics alter genome function to promote increased health and lifespan. *Frontiers in Genetics*, 7, 142.

Guillaumet-Adkins, A., Yañez, Y., Peris-Diaz, M. D., Calabria, I., Palanca-Ballester, C., & Sandoval, J. (2017). Epigenetics and oxidative stress in aging. *Oxidative Medicine and Cellular Longevity*, *2017*.

Guthman, J., & Mansfield, B. (2013). The implications of environmental epigenetics: A new direction for geographic inquiry on health, space, and nature-society relations. *Progress in Human Geography*, *37*(4), 486–504.

Hadacek, F., Bachmann, G., Engelmeier, D., & Chobot, V. (2011). Hormesis and a chemical raison D'être for secondary plant metabolites. *Dose-Response*, *9*(1), 79.

Haiser, H. J., & Turnbaugh, P. J. (2013). Developing a metagenomic view of xenobiotic metabolism. *Pharmacological Research*, *69*(1), 21–31.
Hansen, M., Rubinsztein, D. C., & Walker, D.W. (2018). Autophagy as a promoter of longevity: Insights from model organisms. *Nature Reviews Molecular Cell Biology*, *19*, 579–593.
Henkin, T. M. (2008). Riboswitch RNAs: Using RNA to sense cellular metabolism. *Genes & Development*, *22*(24), 3383–3390.
Holmström, K. M., & Finkel, T. (2014). Cellular mechanisms and physiological consequences of redox-dependent signalling. *Nature Reviews Molecular Cell Biology*, *15*(6), 411.
Ilangumaran, G., & Smith, D. L. (2017). Plant growth promoting rhizobacteria in amelioration of salinity stress: A systems biology perspective. *Frontiers in Plant Science*, *8*, 1768.
Jacobo-Velázquez, D. A., González-Agüero, M., & Cisneros-Zevallos, L. (2015). Cross-talk between signaling pathways: The link between plant secondary metabolite production and wounding stress response. *Scientific Reports*, *5*, 8608.
Jakubowski, W., & Walkowiak, B. (2015). Resistance of oxidative stress in biofilm and planktonic cells. *Brazilian Archives of Biology and Technology*, *58*(2), 300–308.
John, R. M., & Rougeulle, C. (2018). Developmental epigenetics: Phenotype and the flexible epigenome. *Frontiers in Cell and Developmental Biology*, *6*, 130.
Jones, L. M., Rayson, S. J., Flemming, A. J., & Urwin, P. E. (2013). Adaptive and specialised transcriptional responses to xenobiotic stress in Caenorhabditis elegans are regulated by nuclear hormone receptors. *PLoS One*, *8*(7), e69956.
Jones, B. M., & Robinson, G. E. (2018). Genetic accommodation and the role of ancestral plasticity in the evolution of insect eusociality. *Journal of Experimental Biology*, *221*(23), jeb153163.
Kasote, D. M., Katyare, S. S., Hegde, M. V., & Bae, H. (2015). Significance of antioxidant potential of plants and its relevance to therapeutic applications. *International Journal of Biological Sciences*, *11*(8), 982.
Kim, S. M., Hwang, K. A., & Choi, K. C. (2018). Potential roles of reactive oxygen species derived from chemical substances involved in cancer development in the female reproductive system. *BMB Reports*, *51*(11), 557.
Kim, S. A., Lee, Y. M., Choi, J. Y., Jacobs, D. R., Jr., & Lee, D. H. (2018). Evolutionarily adapted hormesis-inducing stressors can be a practical solution to mitigate harmful effects of chronic exposure to low dose chemical mixtures. *Environmental Pollution*, *233*, 725–734.
Koo, H., Allan, R. N., Howlin, R. P., Stoodley, P., & Hall-Stoodley, L. (2017). Targeting microbial biofilms: Current and prospective therapeutic strategies. *Nature Reviews Microbiology*, *15*(12), 740.
Kumar, A., Alam, A., Grover, S., Pandey, S., Tripathi, D., Kumari, M., … Hasnain, S. E. (2019). Peptidyl-prolyl isomerase-B is involved in mycobacterium tuberculosis biofilm formation and a generic target for drug repurposing-based intervention. *NPJ Biofilms and Microbiomes*, *5*(1), 3.
Kuno, T., Hirayama-Kurogi, M., Ito, S., & Ohtsuki, S. (2016). Effect of intestinal flora on protein expression of drug-metabolizing enzymes and transporters in the liver and kidney of germ-free and antibiotics-treated mice. *Molecular Pharmaceutics*, *13*(8), 2691–2701.
Kuno, T., Hirayama-Kurogi, M., Ito, S., & Ohtsuki, S. (2019). Proteomic analysis of small intestinal epithelial cells in antibiotic-treated mice: Changes in drug transporters and metabolizing enzymes. *Drug Metabolism and Pharmacokinetics*, *34*, 159–162.
Kurutas, E. B. (2015). The importance of antioxidants which play the role in cellular response against oxidative/nitrosative stress: Current state. *Nutrition Journal*, *15*(1), 71.
Laforest-Lapointe, I., & Arrieta, M. C. (2018). Microbial eukaryotes: A missing link in gut microbiome studies. *mSystems*, *3*(2). e00201-17.
Lane, P. A. (2018). Ecosystems as chimeras: A thought experiment in Rosennean complexity. *Ecological Complexity*, *35*, 51–75.

Langie, S. A., Koppen, G., Desaulniers, D., Al-Mulla, F., Al-Temaimi, R., Amedei, A., … Charles, A. K. (2015). Causes of genome instability: The effect of low dose chemical exposures in modern society. *Carcinogenesis, 36*(Suppl. 1), S61–S88.
Leak, R. K., Calabrese, E. J., Kozumbo, W. J., Gidday, J. M., Johnson, T. E., Mitchell, J. R., … Bøtker, H. E. (2018). Enhancing and extending biological performance and resilience. *Dose-Response, 16*(3), 1559325818784501.
Lee, H. E., Ayarpadikannan, S., & Kim, H. S. (2016). Role of transposable elements in genomic rearrangement, evolution, gene regulation and epigenetics in primates. *Genes & Genetic Systems*, https://doi.org/10.1266/ggs.15-00016.
Li, C. Y., Lee, S., Cade, S., Kuo, L. J., Schultz, I. R., Bhatt, D. K., … Cui, J. Y. (2017). Novel interactions between gut microbiome and host drug-processing genes modify the hepatic metabolism of the environmental chemicals polybrominated diphenyl ethers. *Drug Metabolism and Disposition, 45*(11), 1197–1214.
Liguori, I., Russo, G., Curcio, F., Bulli, G., Aran, L., Della-Morte, D., … Abete, P. (2018). Oxidative stress, aging, and diseases. *Clinical Interventions in Aging, 13*, 757.
Limborg, M. T., & Heeb, P. (2018). Coevolution of hosts and their microbiome. *Genes, 9*(11).
Lobo, V., Patil, A., Phatak, A., & Chandra, N. (2010). Free radicals, antioxidants and functional foods: Impact on human health. *Pharmacognosy Reviews, 4*(8), 118.
Lomas, P. L., & Giampietro, M. (2017). Environmental accounting for ecosystem conservation: Linking societal and ecosystem metabolisms. *Ecological Modelling, 346*, 10–19.
Lucia, U., & Grisolia, G. (2017). Second law efficiency for living cells. *Frontiers in Bioscience, 9*, 270–275.
Machtel, P., Bąkowska-Żywicka, K., & Żywicki, M. (2016). Emerging applications of riboswitches—From antibacterial targets to molecular tools. *Journal of Applied Genetics, 57*(4), 531–541.
Mansouri, L., Xie, Y., & Rappolee, D. (2012). Adaptive and pathogenic responses to stress by stem cells during development. *Cell, 1*(4), 1197–1224.
Mateo, L., Ullastres, A., & González, J. (2014). A transposable element insertion confers xenobiotic resistance in Drosophila. *PLoS Genetics, 10*(8), e1004560.
Matilainen, O., Quirós, P. M., & Auwerx, J. (2017). Mitochondria and epigenetics—Crosstalk in homeostasis and stress. *Trends in Cell Biology, 27*(6), 453–463.
Medina, A., Schmidt-Heydt, M., Rodriguez, A., Parra, R., Geisen, R., & Magan, N. (2015). Impacts of environmental stress on growth, secondary metabolite biosynthetic gene clusters and metabolite production of xerotolerant/xerophilic fungi. *Current Genetics, 61*(3), 325–334.
Meléndez-Hevia, E., Montero-Gómez, N., & Montero, F. (2008). From prebiotic chemistry to cellular metabolism—The chemical evolution of metabolism before Darwinian natural selection. *Journal of Theoretical Biology, 252*(3), 505–519.
Mhlongo, M. I., Piater, L. A., Madala, N. E., Labuschagne, N., & Dubery, I. A. (2018). The chemistry of plant–microbe interactions in the rhizosphere and the potential for metabolomics to reveal signaling related to defense priming and induced systemic resistance. *Frontiers in Plant Science, 9*, 112.
Milani, C., Duranti, S., Bottacini, F., Casey, E., Turroni, F., Mahony, J., … Lugli, G. A. (2017). The first microbial colonizers of the human gut: Composition, activities, and health implications of the infant gut microbiota. *Microbiology and Molecular Biology Reviews, 81*(4). e00036-17.
Miller, W. (2016). Cognition, information fields and hologenomic entanglement: Evolution in light and shadow. *Biology, 5*(2), 21.
Miller, V. J., Villamena, F. A., & Volek, J. S. (2018). Nutritional ketosis and mitohormesis: Potential implications for mitochondrial function and human health. *Journal of Nutrition and Metabolism, 2018*, 5157645.

Miousse, I. R., Chalbot, M. C. G., Lumen, A., Ferguson, A., Kavouras, I. G., & Koturbash, I. (2015). Response of transposable elements to environmental stressors. *Mutation Research/Reviews in Mutation Research*, *765*, 19–39.
Monteverde, D. R., Sylvan, J. B., Suffridge, C., Baronas, J. J., Fichot, E., Fuhrman, J., … Sañudo-Wilhelmy, S. A. (2018). Distribution of extracellular flavins in a coastal marine basin and their relationship to redox gradients and microbial community members. *Environmental Science & Technology*, *52*(21), 12265–12274.
Muller, A. W. (2005). Thermosynthesis as energy source for the RNA world: A model for the bioenergetics of the origin of life. *Biosystems*, *82*(1), 93–102.
Münger, E., Montiel-Castro, A. J., Langhans, W., & Pacheco-López, G. (2018). Reciprocal interactions between gut microbiota and host social behavior. *Frontiers in Integrative Neuroscience*, *12*, 21.
Naviaux, R. K. (2014). Metabolic features of the cell danger response. *Mitochondrion*, *16*, 7–17.
Naylor, J., Fellermann, H., Ding, Y., Mohammed, W. K., Jakubovics, N. S., Mukherjee, J., … Krasnogor, N. (2017). Simbiotics: A multiscale integrative platform for 3D modeling of bacterial populations. *ACS Synthetic Biology*, *6*(7), 1194–1210.
Nei, M., & Nozawa, M. (2011). Roles of mutation and selection in speciation: From Hugo de Vries to the modern genomic era. *Genome Biology and Evolution*, *3*, 812–829.
Niinemets, Ü., Kahru, A., Mander, Ü., Nõges, P., Nõges, T., Tuvikene, A., & Vasemägi, A. (2017). Interacting environmental and chemical stresses under global change in temperate aquatic ecosystems: Stress responses, adaptation, and scaling. *Regional Environmental Change*, *17*(7), 2061–2077.
Nunn, A. V., Guy, G. W., & Bell, J. D. (2016). The quantum mitochondrion and optimal health. *Biochemical Society Transactions*, *44*(4), 1101–1110.
Nunn, A. V. W., Guy, G. W., & Bell, J. D. (2017). The hormesis of thinking: A deeper quantum thermodynamic perspective? *International Journal of Neurorehabilitation*, *4*(3), 272.
Oh, J., Lee, Y. D., & Wagers, A. J. (2014). Stem cell aging: Mechanisms, regulators and therapeutic opportunities. *Nature Medicine*, *20*(8), 870.
Oliver, K. R., & Greene, W. K. (2011). Mobile DNA and the TE-thrust hypothesis: Supporting evidence from the primates. *Mobile DNA*, *2*(1), 8.
Owusu-Ansah, E., Song, W., & Perrimon, N. (2013). Muscle mitohormesis promotes longevity via systemic repression of insulin signaling. *Cell*, *155*(3), 699–712.
Pandin, C., Le Coq, D., Canette, A., Aymerich, S., & Briandet, R. (2017). Should the biofilm mode of life be taken into consideration for microbial biocontrol agents? *Microbial Biotechnology*, *10*(4), 719–734.
Parashar, A., Gideon, D. A., & Manoj, K. M. (2018). Murburn concept: A molecular explanation for hormetic and idiosyncratic dose responses. *Dose-Response*, *16*(2), 1559325818774421.
Pennisi, M., Crupi, R., Di Paola, R., Ontario, M. L., Bella, R., Calabrese, E. J., … Calabrese, V. (2017). Inflammasomes, hormesis, and antioxidants in neuroinflammation: Role of NRLP3 in Alzheimer disease. *Journal of Neuroscience Research*, *95*(7), 1360–1372.
Picard, M., McEwen, B. S., Epel, E. S., & Sandi, C. (2018). An energetic view of stress: Focus on mitochondria. *Frontiers in Neuroendocrinology*, *49*, 72–85.
Poljsak, B. (2011). Strategies for reducing or preventing the generation of oxidative stress. *Oxidative Medicine and Cellular Longevity*, *2011*.
Postler, T. S., & Ghosh, S. (2017). Understanding the holobiont: How microbial metabolites affect human health and shape the immune system. *Cell Metabolism*, *26*(1), 110–130.
Prasad, R., Shah, A. H., & Dhamgaye, S. (2014). *Mechanisms of drug resistance in fungi and their significance in biofilms*. In *Antibiofilm agents*. Berlin, Heidelberg: Springer. (pp. 45–65).
Racchi, M. (2013). Antioxidant defenses in plants with attention to Prunus and Citrus spp. *Antioxidants*, *2*(4), 340–369.

Rahal, A., Kumar, A., Singh, V., Yadav, B., Tiwari, R., Chakraborty, S., & Dhama, K. (2014). Oxidative stress, prooxidants, and antioxidants: The interplay. *BioMed Research International, 2014.*

Rattan, S. I. (2012). Rationale and methods of discovering hormetins as drugs for healthy ageing. *Expert Opinion on Drug Discovery*, 7(5), 439–448.

Rattan, S. I. (2014). Aging is not a disease: Implications for intervention. *Aging and Disease, 5*(3), 196.

Rattan, S. I., Sejersen, H., Fernandes, R. A., & Luo, W. (2007). Stress-mediated hormetic modulation of aging, wound healing, and angiogenesis in human cells. *Annals of the New York Academy of Sciences, 1119*(1), 112–121.

Razeto-Barry, P. (2012). Autopoiesis 40 years later. A review and a reformulation. *Origins of Life and Evolution of Biospheres, 42*(6), 543–567.

Restivo, S. (2018). *Kingdom of the crystal myth: Love and evolution.* In *The age of the social.* Routledge. (pp. 108–131).

Ristow, M., & Schmeisser, K. (2014). Mitohormesis: Promoting health and lifespan by increased levels of reactive oxygen species (ROS). *Dose-Response, 12*(2), 288.

Rodriguez, M., Snoek, L. B., Riksen, J. A., Bevers, R. P., & Kammenga, J. E. (2012). Genetic variation for stress-response hormesis in C. elegans lifespan. *Experimental Gerontology, 47*(8), 581–587.

Römling, U., & Balsalobre, C. (2012). Biofilm infections, their resilience to therapy and innovative treatment strategies. *Journal of Internal Medicine, 272*(6), 541–561.

Salvioli, A., Ghignone, S., Novero, M., Navazio, L., Bagnaresi, P., & Bonfante, P. (2016). Symbiosis with an endobacterium increases the fitness of a mycorrhizal fungus, raising its bioenergetic potential. *The ISME Journal, 10*(1), 130.

Schieber, M., & Chandel, N. S. (2014). ROS function in redox signaling and oxidative stress. *Current Biology, 24*(10), R453–R462.

Scott, B. R. (2014). Radiation-hormesis phenotypes, the related mechanisms and implications for disease prevention and therapy. *Journal of Cell Communication and Signaling, 8*(4), 341–352.

Segré, D., Shenhav, B., Kafri, R., & Lancet, D. (2001). The molecular roots of compositional inheritance. *Journal of Theoretical Biology, 213*(3), 481–491.

Segref, A., Kevei, E., Pokrzywa, W., Schmeisser, K., Mansfeld, J., Livnat-Levanon, N., ... Hoppe, T. (2014). Pathogenesis of human mitochondrial diseases is modulated by reduced activity of the ubiquitin/proteasome system. *Cell Metabolism, 19*(4), 642–652.

Shadel, G. S., & Horvath, T. L. (2015). Mitochondrial ROS signaling in organismal homeostasis. *Cell, 163*(3), 560–569.

Sharma, P., Jha, A. B., Dubey, R. S., & Pessarakli, M. (2012). Reactive oxygen species, oxidative damage, and antioxidative defense mechanism in plants under stressful conditions. *Journal of Botany, 2012.*

Shimi, T., & Goldman, R. D. (2014). *Nuclear lamins and oxidative stress in cell proliferation and longevity.* In *Cancer biology and the nuclear envelope.* New York, NY: Springer. (pp. 415–430).

Sies, H. (2019). Oxidative stress: Eustress and distress in redox homeostasis. In G. Fink (Ed.), *Stress: Physiology, biochemistry, and pathology* (pp. 153–163). USA: Academic Press.

Simon, J. C., Marchesi, J. R., Mougel, C., & Selosse, M. A. (2019). Host-microbiota interactions: From holobiont theory to analysis. *Microbiome*, 7(1), 5.

Siriwardena, A. K. (2014). Reappraisal of xenobiotic-induced, oxidative stress-mediated cellular injury in chronic pancreatitis: A systematic review. *World Journal of Gastroenterology: WJG, 20*(11), 3033.

Slaveykova, V., Sonntag, B., & Gutiérrez, J. C. (2016). Stress and protists: No life without stress. *European Journal of Protistology, 55*, 39–49.

Solleiro-Villavicencio, H., & Rivas-Arancibia, S. (2018). Effect of chronic oxidative stress on neuroinflammatory response mediated by CD4+ T cells in neurodegenerative diseases. *Frontiers in Cellular Neuroscience*, *12*, 114.

Son, J. M., & Lee, C. (2019). Mitochondria: Multifaceted regulators of aging. *BMB Reports*, *52*(1), 13.

Spanogiannopoulos, P., Bess, E. N., Carmody, R. N., & Turnbaugh, P. J. (2016). The microbial pharmacists within us: A metagenomic view of xenobiotic metabolism. *Nature Reviews Microbiology*, *14*(5), 273.

Spooner, R., & Yilmaz, Ö. (2011). The role of reactive-oxygen-species in microbial persistence and inflammation. *International Journal of Molecular Sciences*, *12*(1), 334–352.

Stockhorst, U., & Antov, M. I. (2016). Modulation of fear extinction by stress, stress hormones and estradiol: A review. *Frontiers in Behavioral Neuroscience*, *9*, 359.

Stotz, K., & Allen, C. (2012). From cell-surface receptors to higher learning: A whole world of experience. In K. Plaisance & T. Reydom (Eds.), *Philosophy of behavioral biology* (pp. 85–123). Dordrecht: Springer.

Suliman, H. B., & Piantadosi, C. A. (2016). Mitochondrial quality control as a therapeutic target. *Pharmacological Reviews*, *68*(1), 20–48.

Swinnen, E., Ghillebert, R., Wilms, T., & Winderickx, J. (2014). Molecular mechanisms linking the evolutionary conserved TORC1-Sch9 nutrient signalling branch to lifespan regulation in *Saccharomyces cerevisiae*. *FEMS Yeast Research*, *14*(1), 17–32.

Tan, H. Y., Wang, N., Li, S., Hong, M., Wang, X., & Feng, Y. (2016). The reactive oxygen species in macrophage polarization: Reflecting its dual role in progression and treatment of human diseases. *Oxidative Medicine and Cellular Longevity*, *2016*.

Tizioto, P. C., Coutinho, L. L., Oliveira, P. S., Cesar, A. S., Diniz, W. J., Lima, A. O., … Tullio, R. R. (2016). Gene expression differences in longissimus muscle of Nelore steers genetically divergent for residual feed intake. *Scientific Reports*, *6*, 39493.

Tripathy, B. C., & Oelmüller, R. (2012). Reactive oxygen species generation and signaling in plants. *Plant Signaling & Behavior*, 7(12), 1621–1633.

Vaiserman, A. M. (2010). Hormesis, adaptive epigenetic reorganization, and implications for human health and longevity. *Dose-Response*, *8*(1), 16.

Vaiserman, A. M. (2011). Hormesis and epigenetics: Is there a link? *Ageing Research Reviews*, *10*(4), 413–421.

Valero, T. (2014). Editorial (thematic issue: Mitochondrial biogenesis: Pharmacological approaches). *Current Pharmaceutical Design*, *20*(35), 5507–5509.

Vargas-Hernandez, M., Macias-Bobadilla, I., Guevara-Gonzalez, R. G., Romero-Gomez, S. D. J., Rico-Garcia, E., Ocampo-Velazquez, R. V., … Torres-Pacheco, I. (2017). Plant hormesis management with biostimulants of biotic origin in agriculture. *Frontiers in Plant Science*, *8*, 1762.

Varriale, A. (2014). DNA methylation, epigenetics, and evolution in vertebrates: Facts and challenges. *International Journal of Evolutionary Biology*, *2014*.

Villa, F., Cappitelli, F., Cortesi, P., & Kunova, A. (2017). Fungal biofilms: Targets for the development of novel strategies in plant disease management. *Frontiers in Microbiology*, *8*, 654.

Wallace, R., & Wallace, D. (2009). Code, context, and epigenetic catalysis in gene expression. In C. Priami (Ed.), *Transactions on computational systems biology XI* (pp. 283–334). Berlin, Heidelberg: Springer.

Weis, J. S. (2012). Evolution in a toxic world: How life responds to chemical threats. *Bioscience*, *62*(12), 1086–1088.

Wu, H. J., & Wu, E. (2012). The role of gut microbiota in immune homeostasis and autoimmunity. *Gut Microbes*, *3*(1), 4–14.

Yun, J., & Finkel, T. (2014). Mitohormesis. *Cell Metabolism*, *19*(5), 757–766.

Zengler, K. (2009). Central role of the cell in microbial ecology. *Microbiology and Molecular Biology Reviews*, *73*(4), 712–729.
Zheng, Y., Zhao, X., Jia, K., Li, J., Wang, L., Wang, R., ... Zhang, D. (2018). bifA regulates biofilm development of Pseudomonas putida MnB1 as a primary response to H2O2 and Mn2+. *Frontiers in Microbiology*, *9*, 1490.
Zivieri, R., Pacini, N., Finocchio, G., & Carpentieri, M. (2017). Rate of entropy model for irreversible processes in living systems. *Scientific Reports*, 7(1), 9134.
Zorov, D. B., Juhaszova, M., & Sollott, S. J. (2014). Mitochondrial reactive oxygen species (ROS) and ROS-induced ROS release. *Physiological Reviews*, *94*(3), 909–950.

Further reading

Calabrese, E. J., & Mattson, M. P. (2017). How does hormesis impact biology, toxicology, and medicine? *NPJ Aging and Mechanisms of Disease*, *3*(1), 13.

CHAPTER 9

Autocatakinesis systems in drug discovery

Organic life, we are told, has developed gradually from the protozoon to the philosopher, and this development, we are assured, is indubitably an advance. Unfortunately it is the philosopher, not the protozoon, who gives us this assurance.

An extra-terrestrial philosopher, who had watched a single youth up to the age of twenty-one and had never come across any other human being, might conclude that it is the nature of human beings to grow continually taller and wiser in an indefinite progress towards perfection; and this generalization would be just as well founded as the generalization which evolutionists base upon the previous history of this planet.

We have reached a stage in evolution which is not the final stage. We must pass through it quickly, for if we do not, most of us will perish by the way, and the others will be lost in a forest of doubt and fear. Envy therefore, evil as it is, and terrible as are its effects, is not wholly of the devil. It is in part the expression of a heroic pain, the pain of those who walk through the night blindly, perhaps to a better resting-place, perhaps only to death and destruction. To find the right road out of this despair civilised man must enlarge his heart as he has enlarged his mind. He must learn to transcend self, and in so doing to acquire the freedom of the Universe.

Bertrand Russell (1872–1970)

9.1 Introduction

An autocatakinetic system represents an auto-ordered system that interacts with its environment to share entropy (Baggs & Chemero, 2018; Plasson et al., 2015; Swenson, 1997); this self-organized system allows the development of autocatalytic reactions for the self-production of the living system and thus establish the molecular metabolic networks necessary to obtain

Molecular Evolutionary Models in Drug Discovery
https://doi.org/10.1016/B978-0-12-817613-9.00009-2

energy from the nutrients and proliferate (Hordijk, 2016; Hordijk & Steel, 2017, 2018). Thus, any biological system that acquires autocatakinetic capacity develops complex metabolic pathways for the optimization of the use of energy and, therefore, requires a chemically diverse secondary metabolism that allows the proper functioning of the primary metabolism (Hill, Czauderna, Klapperstück, Roessner, & Schreiber, 2015; Metallo & Vander Heiden, 2013; Pröschel, Detsch, Boccaccini, & Sonnewald, 2015). Likewise, molecular signaling networks allow the self-organization and regulation of entropy within the biological system, so that molecular evolution has been largely directed by negentropy (Fig. 1) (Davies, Rieper, & Tuszynski, 2013; Lancet, Zidovetzki, & Markovitch, 2018; Torday, 2016). Equally, thermodynamic equilibrium and homeostasis are the bases on which the functionality of the innovations of chemical evolution are determined (Davidi, Longo, Jabłońska, Milo, & Tawfik, 2018; Davies & Walker, 2016; Moreno, 2016).

Thus, the maintenance of autocatakinesis acquires importance insofar as it sustains the functional structure of biological systems, which is necessary for the development of coevolution, symbiosis, and communication between individuals in an ecosystem (Berlanga, 2015; Vijver, Salthe, & Delpos, 2013). This change in structure and function is only consolidated in the acquisition of fitness by the system, so in this way the functionality allows the energy reactions and the sharing of information and entropy (Jha & Udgaonkar, 2010; Lucia, 2015; Yufik, 2019). Additionally, the

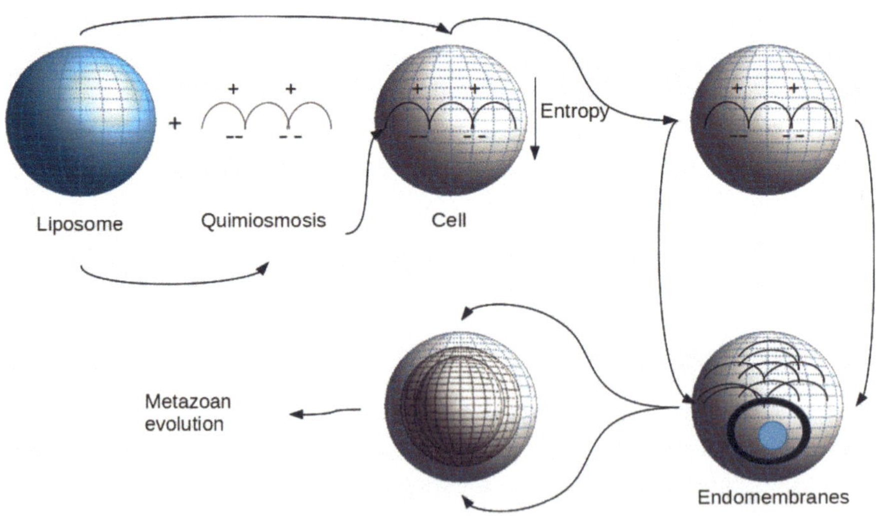

Fig. 1 Evolution of form and function by virtue of entropy and homeostasis.

disease is a product of the disruption of self-organization as well as the metabolic pathways responsible for maintaining the functionality of the system (DeBerardinis & Thompson, 2012; Ito & Suda, 2014; MacIver, Michalek, & Rathmell, 2013). Thus, a new pharmacological approach must be capable of restoring the self-organization capacities of the biological systems affected by the metabolic disorder and restoring the interaction and communication networks that lead to homeostasis (Brestoff & Artis, 2015; Goldman et al., 2015; Silverman & Deuster, 2014). For these reasons, the objective of this chapter is to analyze autocatakinesis as a metabolic model of health and disease with which to develop new pharmacological applications that allow patients to survive and acquire fitness (Marijuán, Navarro, & del Moral, 2015; Plasson, Brandenburg, Jullien, & Bersini, 2011; Swenson, 1997).

9.2 Metabolic autocatakinesis

Metabolic autocatakinesis represents the self-organization of metabolic networks that allow the autopoiesis of the biological system to be open in interaction and communication with its ecosystem (Marijuán, Navarro, & del Moral, 2010; Moral, González, Navarro, & Marijuán, 2011; Swenson, 1992). So this metabolic phenomenon as a model allows us to calculate the sharing of entropy between the individuals of the biological system that leads to energy homeostasis (Cannon, 2014; Recordati & Bellini, 2004; Vallino, 2010). In this way, life could be established by reaching a thermodynamic equilibrium with its environment in association with other individuals (Matsuno, 2017; Wei, Xi, Nussinov, & Ma, 2016; Wosniack, da Luz, & Schulman, 2017). Likewise, these thermodynamic fluctuations in the search for equilibrium determined the associations and configurations of the proteins as well as the chemical association signals that the proto-cells produced (Bronowska, 2011; Danielsson et al., 2015; Díaz-Villanueva, Díaz-Molina, & García-González, 2015). Additionally, thermodynamic self-organization promoted the symbiotic association between species and groups through the chemical signals of secondary metabolism, as happened with biofilms as a model of polymicrobial mutualism (Chavez-Dozal & Nishiguchi, 2011; Foster & Bell, 2012; Rickard et al., 2006). Likewise, thermodynamic self-organization becomes a driver of chemical diversity by promoting the functionality and optimization of metabolic pathways as the basis for adaptation and fitness acquisition (Egel, 2012; Na, Kim, & Lee, 2010; Scirè & Annovazzi-Lodi, 2017). So when the autocatakinesis metabolic is possible, self-replicating molecules make the biological system become autopoietic, and thus, the information acquired in the cognition of responding to environmental stress can be passed on to the next generation (Bitbol & Luisi, 2004; Dollens, 2015; Letelier, Marın, & Mpodozis, 2003).

On the other hand, it must be taken into account that the adaptive responses to stress mediated by reactive oxygen species (ROS) must be part of the metabolic self-organization by allowing the system to acquire greater functionality in obtaining energy and competition for space (Espinosa-Diez et al., 2015; Kurutas, 2015; Zorov, Juhaszova, & Sollott, 2014). In this adaptive response, functional phenotypic changes are acquired under autocatakinesis; in addition, the regulation of gene expression is activated in the search for greater functionality and optimization of metabolic pathways to obtain energy (Bathe & Farshidfar, 2014; Chubukov, Zuleta, & Li, 2012; Metallo & Vander Heiden, 2013). The gene expression of the enzymes in the biosynthetic pathways is thermodynamically modulated, as well as their structural changes depending on the environmental stress, all in function of allowing the utilization of the nutrients and the survival (Genereux & Wiseman, 2015; Hauryliuk, Atkinson, Murakami, Tenson, & Gerdes, 2015; Liu, Li, Liu, & Cao, 2013). In the same way, the form and mobility of living organisms has been modified by the metabolic sharing of entropy, in order to reach the sources of energy and be able to find spaces to prosper (Baum, 2018; Danchin, 2018; Kirchhoff & Froese, 2017). Thus, important phenomena for cell survival, such as chemotaxis and cell recognition, have been developed due to self-organization to cope with environmental and nutritional changes (Ildefonso, 2015; Kurakin, 2011; Lefevre et al., 2017). Finally, this evolutionary model is determined by proteostasis and self-organization in thermodynamic equilibrium (Caetano-Anollés, Wang, Caetano-Anollés, & Mittenthal, 2009; Hoelzer, Smith, & Pepper, 2006; Ramakrishnan, Houben, Rousseau, & Schymkowitz, 2019).

9.3 The RNA world, proteostasis, and thermodynamic equilibrium

Protein homeostasis, or proteostasis, was achieved when the protein world was self-organized by the RNA world, which is considered an important step in the establishment of a functional cellular system (Caetano-Anollés & Seufferheld, 2013; Gomez-Verjan, Vazquez-Martinez, Rivero-Segura, & Medina-Campos, 2018; Powers & Balch, 2013). Thus, the RNA world increased the functionality of the protein world by making the molecular information required to establish the different biosynthetic pathways mediated by enzymes self-replicating (Chatterjee & Yadav, 2019; Saad, 2018;

Yarus, 2011). This self-organization capacity that is acquired when the RNA world replicates the information for the maintenance of homeostasis allows the establishment of the initial Darwinian ancestor (IDA), which is prior to the universal common ancestor (LUCA) (Domagal-Goldman et al., 2016; Glansdorff, Xu, & Labedan, 2008; Hoenigsberg, 2003). Likewise, LUCA requires optimal metabolic pathways in equilibrium, which allow the sharing of entropy, so that biosynthetic pathways as they interact undergo modifications to achieve chemical diversity (Alam-Nazki & Krishnan, 2015; Braakman & Smith, 2012a, 2012b). In this way, the riboswitches and coenzymes nicotinamide adenine dinucleotide (NAD^+) and flavin adenine dinucleotide (FAD^+) that catalyze oxidoreduction reactions were a fundamental part in regulating protein synthesis and its modifications to obtain metabolic pathways with greater functionality to consolidate proteostasis in the RNA world (Batey, 2012; Vitreschak, Rodionov, Mironov, & Gelfand, 2004; Yang & Sauve, 2016).

However, it is important to keep in mind that proteostasis is possible to the extent that metabolic pathways are more efficient in the sharing of entropy; that means functionality (Chan, Zhang, Wallin, & Liu, 2011; Powers, Morimoto, Dillin, Kelly, & Balch, 2009; Wolynes, 2015), and that functionality is associated with the folding of proteins, then chaperones enter to play an important role in the reactivity of enzymes that allow the thermodynamic equilibrium of the biological system (Braakman & Hebert, 2013; Ikwegbue, Masamba, Oyinloye, & Kappo, 2018; Vabulas, Raychaudhuri, Hayer-Hartl, & Hartl, 2010). This is how heat shock proteins (Hsp) become an important mechanism that drives the coevolution between metabolites and enzymes as well as self-organization in the initial biological system controlled by the RNA world (Maleki, Afra Khosravi, Taghinejad, & Azizian, 2016; Park & Seo, 2015; Saibil, 2013). Thus Hsp help the synthesis and diversity of catalytic proteins in response to environmental stress, allowing the adaptation and innovation of biosynthetic pathways, leading to molecular evolution (Jarosz & Lindquist, 2010; Pan, 2013; Storey & Wu, 2013). In this way, the response to stress mediated by Hsp drives proteostasis in the search for balance and maintains the structure and self-organization of the biological system (Di Domenico, Head, Butterfield, & Perluigi, 2014; Klaips, Jayaraj, & Hartl, 2018; Labbadia & Morimoto, 2015).

9.4 Heat shock proteins, adaptative response, and thermodynamic evolution

The response to stress mediated by Hsp allows the acquisition of fitness by modifying the folding of the synthesized proteins in order to increase the enzymatic promiscuity, achieve an optimization of the metabolic networks, and obtain greater energy from the available sources (Evans, Chang, & Gestwicki, 2010; Fares, 2014; Lee, Chao, Cheng, & Leu, 2018). So Hsp maintains self-organization so that self-replicating molecules can transmit information and disseminate proteostasis pathways (Dong & Cui, 2019; Latorre, Mattenberger, & Geller, 2018; Yerbury et al., 2016). Likewise, protein stability in response to stress is important during initial phenotypic adaptations, which makes Hsp an epigenetic expression regulation factor that prevents damage to the cellular machinery and promotes the acquisition of fitness (Horowitz, 2015; Migicovsky, Yao, & Kovalchuk, 2014; Moradali, Ghods, & Rehm, 2017). So, Hsp in the RNA world evolved as a mechanism to defend the information encoded to prevent it from being degraded by environmental changes (Fulda, Gorman, Hori, & Samali, 2010; Wang, Vinocur, Shoseyov, & Altman, 2004; Wei & Murphy, 2016). This is observed in the protection of the splicing of mRNA carried out by heat shock proteins in the presence of heat, in order to maintain proteostasis (Fujimoto & Nakai, 2010; Shalgi, Hurt, Lindquist, & Burge, 2014; Verghese, Abrams, Wang, & Morano, 2012). Likewise, this response to heat promotes the production of secondary metabolites mediated by Hsp that increases the thermotolerance (Ghasemi, Jelodar, Modarresi, & Bagheri, 2013; Qu, Ding, Jiang, & Zhu, 2013; Wahid, Gelani, Ashraf, & Foolad, 2007).

Thus, the chemically diverse compounds induced by heat shock proteins will allow both cell survival and transmission of proteostasis to other individuals in the biological system (Lindquist & Kelly, 2011; Takeuchi et al., 2015; Triandafillou, Katanski, Dinner, & Drummond, 2018). Then the heat shock response (HSR) as a whole corresponds to a mechanism of transcriptional regulation that is part of the set of phenotypic adaptations, and acquiring functionality by allowing homeostasis causes the modifications to be inherited (Amaral, Dinger, & Mattick, 2013; Maresca & Schwartz, 2006; Morano, Grant, & Moye-Rowley, 2012). Equally, by inheriting the adaptive changes for survival, these are maintained as long as the environmental stress persists, so the Hsp are also a source of phenotypic plasticity in the coevolution and speciation (Gilbert, Bosch, & Ledón-Rettig, 2015; Kaneko & Furusawa, 2018; Soen, Knafo, & Elgart, 2015). Finally, an autocatakinetic system that maintains its functional structure in adaptation and survival through the protection of its protein balance can enter into communication with other systems to form signaling networks with which to establish symbiotic communities of exchange (Nousala, 2012; Swenson, 1998).

9.5 Autocatakinesis, symbiosis, interactions, and balance in mutualism

A symbiotic relationship between self-organized systems grows in the exchange of entropy and communication, thus achieving a synergism that allows individuals to achieve homeostasis (Abel, 2009; Corning, 1995; Torday, 2015). In this way, the signaling molecules that are produced to expand the proteostasis of the system promote thermodynamic equilibrium by distributing adaptive information, such as hormones (Mardones, Martínez, & Hetz, 2015; van Oosten-Hawle & Morimoto, 2014; van Oosten-Hawle, Porter, & Morimoto, 2013). Then, in a symbiotic system such as the holobiont, self-organization should have a thermodynamic equilibrium among all individuals in order to establish the molecular networks that make it up (Ivanitskii, 2017; Miller, 2016; Root-Bernstein & Dillon, 1997). This is how eukaryotic life emerged as a holobiont, being in endosymbiosis, and how it becomes more complex among the species with which it establishes mutualism (Aanen & Eggleton, 2017; Bordenstein & Theis, 2015; O'Malley, 2015). In these complex systems, communication networks are established to acquire cognition of the surrounding environment; this is where the hormetic response mediated by reactive oxygen species (ROS) and the adaptive heat response mediated by Hsp aided in the formation of metabolic networks for obtaining and sharing energy (Calabrese et al., 2011; Mao & Franke, 2013; Zimmermann, Bauer, Kroemer, Madeo, & Carmona-Gutierrez, 2014). In this way, the disruption of the symbiosis originates in a loss of self-organization and this leads to the alteration of the metabolic networks in the system that leads to disease (Belkaid & Hand, 2014; Porporato, Filigheddu, Bravo-San Pedro, Kroemer, & Galluzzi, 2018; Round & Mazmanian, 2009). Thus, the dysbiosis as an alteration of the microbial populations in the holobiont is promoted in the metabolic modifications resulting from the loss of self-organization (Lachnit, Bosch, & Deines, 2019; Pita, Rix, Slaby, Franke, & Hentschel, 2018; Webster & Thomas, 2016). Finally, both symbiotic and metabolic disruption induces the alteration of the hologenome, which confers diminution of the adaptive capacity to the system and increases its disorder (Jovel, Dieleman, Kao, Mason, & Wine, 2018; Muraille, 2018; West, Jenmalm, & Prescott, 2015).

9.6 Autocatakinesis systems in drug discovery

Maintaining the self-organization of the biological system is necessary to achieve homeostasis in the health-disease duality (Kotas & Medzhitov, 2015; Seeley, 2002). This can be achieved by restoring altered metabolic networks, as well as interrupted symbiosis and proteostasis of the biological system (Gorgoulis, Pefani, Pateras, & Trougakos, 2018; Maguire & Maguire, 2019). Thus, the modulation of thermal stress proteins such as Hsp becomes an adequate therapeutic target to reduce the disorder of the system and restore homeostasis (Dattilo et al., 2015; West, Wang, & Morano, 2012; Zuo, Subjeck, & Wang, 2016). Likewise, proteostasis becomes an adaptive factor in an attractive therapeutic target for degenerative diseases, cancer, and infections (Calamini & Morimoto, 2012; Lupoli, Vaubourgeix, Burns-Huang, & Gold, 2018; Mercado & Hetz, 2017). The reestablishment of the proteostasis network allows recovery of normal physiology by means of two pharmacological approaches: the synthesis and use of the Hsp as medicines, and the prevention of the degradation of the physiological components of the network by means of small molecules (Bouchecareilh, Conkright, & Balch, 2010; Hipp, Kasturi, & Hartl, 2019; Maiuri, Raia, & Kroemer, 2017). In this way, the maintenance of the proteostasis will boost the stability of the self-organization and, therefore, the nature of the symbiosis that makes up the holobiont (Hurst, 2017; Mao & Franke, 2015). Therefore, any pharmacological model of impact must take the biological system to its state of thermodynamic equilibrium in order to achieve an optimal cure (Copeland, 2016; Garbett & Chaires, 2012).

9.7 Conclusions

Self-organized biological systems allow the establishment of metabolic networks where the proliferation and interaction of individuals is possible (Saetzler, Sonnenschein, & Soto, 2011; Somvanshi & Venkatesh, 2014). In this way, self-organization depends on the maintenance of the functional structure of the system that is carried out through proteostasis (Gorenberg & Chandra, 2017). Likewise, chaperones as heat shock proteins represent a mechanism that allows homeostasis and the protection of cellular functions (Stetler et al., 2010); these heat shock proteins were fundamental in the protection of RNA in the proto-cell and promoted the dissemination of proteostasis by establishing networks of communication and interaction in cell communities (Demirsoy, Martin, Maes, & Agostinis, 2016). For this reason, autocatakinetic systems are attractive models for the development of new therapeutic targets that seek to restore lost proteostasis or decrease the operational functional structure of diseases such as cancer. In addition, self-organizing systems are a cornerstone of metabolic networks sharing energy, which also makes them promising for the design of new drugs and personalized nutrition protocols for the treatment of metabolic disorders (de Toro-Martín, Arsenault, Després, & Vohl, 2017).

References

Aanen, D. K., & Eggleton, P. (2017). Symbiogenesis: Beyond the endosymbiosis theory? *Journal of Theoretical Biology*, *434*, 99–103.

Abel, D. (2009). The capabilities of chaos and complexity. *International Journal of Molecular Sciences*, *10*(1), 247–291.

Alam-Nazki, A., & Krishnan, J. (2015). Spatial control of biochemical modification cascades and pathways. *Biophysical Journal*, *108*(12), 2912–2924.

Amaral, P. P., Dinger, M. E., & Mattick, J. S. (2013). Non-coding RNAs in homeostasis, disease and stress responses: An evolutionary perspective. *Briefings in Functional Genomics*, *12*(3), 254–278.

Baggs, E., & Chemero, A. (2018). Radical embodiment in two directions. *Synthese*, 1–16.

Batey, R. T. (2012). Structure and mechanism of purine-binding riboswitches. *Quarterly Reviews of Biophysics*, *45*(3), 345–381.

Bathe, O., & Farshidfar, F. (2014). From genotype to functional phenotype: Unraveling the metabolomic features of colorectal cancer. *Genes*, *5*(3), 536–560.

Baum, D. A. (2018). The origin and early evolution of life in chemical composition space. *Journal of Theoretical Biology*, *456*, 295–304.

Belkaid, Y., & Hand, T. W. (2014). Role of the microbiota in immunity and inflammation. *Cell*, *157*(1), 121–141.

Berlanga, M. (2015). Functional symbiosis and communication in microbial ecosystems. The case of wood-eating termites and cockroaches. *International Microbiology*, *18*(3), 159–169.

Bitbol, M., & Luisi, P. L. (2004). Autopoiesis with or without cognition: Defining life at its edge. *Journal of the Royal Society Interface*, *1*(1), 99–107.

Bordenstein, S. R., & Theis, K. R. (2015). Host biology in light of the microbiome: Ten principles of holobionts and hologenomes. *PLoS Biology*, *13*(8), e1002226.

Bouchecareilh, M., Conkright, J. J., & Balch, W. E. (2010). Proteostasis strategies for restoring α1-antitrypsin deficiency. *Proceedings of the American Thoracic Society*, 7(6), 415–422.

Braakman, I., & Hebert, D. N. (2013). Protein folding in the endoplasmic reticulum. *Cold Spring Harbor Perspectives in Biology*, *5*(5), a013201.

Braakman, R., & Smith, E. (2012a). The compositional and evolutionary logic of metabolism. *Physical Biology*, *10*(1), 011001.

Braakman, R., & Smith, E. (2012b). The emergence and early evolution of biological carbon-fixation. *PLoS Computational Biology*, *8*(4), e1002455.

Brestoff, J. R., & Artis, D. (2015). Immune regulation of metabolic homeostasis in health and disease. *Cell*, *161*(1), 146–160.

Bronowska, A. K. (2011). Thermodynamics of ligand-protein interactions: Implications for molecular design. In J. C. Moreno (Ed.), *Thermodynamics-interaction studies-solids, liquids and gases* (pp. 1–48). London: IntechOpen.

Caetano-Anollés, G., & Seufferheld, M. J. (2013). The coevolutionary roots of biochemistry and cellular organization challenge the RNA world paradigm. *Journal of Molecular Microbiology and Biotechnology*, *23*(1–2), 152–177.

Caetano-Anollés, G., Wang, M., Caetano-Anollés, D., & Mittenthal, J. E. (2009). The origin, evolution and structure of the protein world. *Biochemical Journal*, *417*(3), 621–637.

Calabrese, V., Cornelius, C., Cuzzocrea, S., Iavicoli, I., Rizzarelli, E., & Calabrese, E. J. (2011). Hormesis, cellular stress response and vitagenes as critical determinants in aging and longevity. *Molecular Aspects of Medicine*, *32*(4–6), 279–304.

Calamini, B., & Morimoto, R. I. (2012). Protein homeostasis as a therapeutic target for diseases of protein conformation. *Current Topics in Medicinal Chemistry*, *12*(22), 2623–2640.

Cannon, W. R. (2014). Concepts, challenges, and successes in modeling thermodynamics of metabolism. *Frontiers in Bioengineering and Biotechnology*, *2*, 53.

Chan, H. S., Zhang, Z., Wallin, S., & Liu, Z. (2011). Cooperativity, local-nonlocal coupling, and nonnative interactions: Principles of protein folding from coarse-grained models. *Annual Review of Physical Chemistry*, *62*, 301–326.
Chatterjee, S., & Yadav, S. (2019). The origin of prebiotic information system in the peptide/ RNA world: A simulation model of the evolution of translation and the genetic code. *Life*, *9*(1), 25.
Chavez-Dozal, A., & Nishiguchi, M. K. (2011). Variation in biofilm formation among symbiotic and free-living strains of *Vibrio fischeri*. *Journal of Basic Microbiology*, *51*(5), 452–458.
Chubukov, V., Zuleta, I. A., & Li, H. (2012). Regulatory architecture determines optimal regulation of gene expression in metabolic pathways. *Proceedings of the National Academy of Sciences*, *109*(13), 5127–5132.
Copeland, R. A. (2016). The drug–target residence time model: A 10-year retrospective. *Nature Reviews Drug Discovery*, *15*(2), 87.
Corning, P. A. (1995). Synergy and self-organization in the evolution of complex systems. *Systems Research*, *12*(2), 89–121.
Danchin, A. (2018). *Multiple clocks in the evolution of living organisms*. In *Molecular mechanisms of microbial evolution*. Cham: Springer. (pp. 101–118).
Danielsson, J., Mu, X., Lang, L., Wang, H., Binolfi, A., Theillet, F. X., ... Oliveberg, M. (2015). Thermodynamics of protein destabilization in live cells. *Proceedings of the National Academy of Sciences*, *112*(40), 12402–12407.
Dattilo, S., Mancuso, C., Koverech, G., Di Mauro, P., Ontario, M. L., Petralia, C. C., ... Calabrese, V. (2015). Heat shock proteins and hormesis in the diagnosis and treatment of neurodegenerative diseases. *Immunity & Ageing*, *12*(1), 20.
Davidi, D., Longo, L. M., Jabłońska, J., Milo, R., & Tawfik, D. S. (2018). A bird's-eye view of enzyme evolution: Chemical, physicochemical, and physiological considerations. *Chemical Reviews*, *118*(18), 8786–8797.
Davies, P. C., Rieper, E., & Tuszynski, J. A. (2013). Self-organization and entropy reduction in a living cell. *Biosystems*, *111*(1), 1–10.
Davies, P. C., & Walker, S. I. (2016). The hidden simplicity of biology. *Reports on Progress in Physics*, *79*(10), 102601.
de Toro-Martín, J., Arsenault, B., Després, J. P., & Vohl, M. C. (2017). Precision nutrition: A review of personalized nutritional approaches for the prevention and management of metabolic syndrome. *Nutrients*, *9*(8), 913.
DeBerardinis, R. J., & Thompson, C. B. (2012). Cellular metabolism and disease: What do metabolic outliers teach us? *Cell*, *148*(6), 1132–1144.
Demirsoy, S., Martin, S., Maes, H., & Agostinis, P. (2016). Adapt, recycle, and move on: Proteostasis and trafficking mechanisms in melanoma. *Frontiers in Oncology*, *6*, 240.
Di Domenico, F., Head, E., Butterfield, D. A., & Perluigi, M. (2014). Oxidative stress and proteostasis network: Culprit and casualty of Alzheimer's-like neurodegeneration. *Advances in Geriatrics*, *2014*.
Díaz-Villanueva, J., Díaz-Molina, R., & García-González, V. (2015). Protein folding and mechanisms of proteostasis. *International Journal of Molecular Sciences*, *16*(8), 17193–17230.
Dollens, D. (2015). Autopoiesis+ extended cognition+ nature= can buildings think? *Communicative & Integrative Biology*, *8*(4), e994373.
Domagal-Goldman, S. D., Wright, K. E., Adamala, K., Arina de la Rubia, L., Bond, J., Dartnell, L. R., ... Singer, K. (2016). The astrobiology primer v2.0. *Astrobiology*, *16*(8), 561–653.
Dong, Z., & Cui, H. (2019). The autophagy-lysosomal pathways and their emerging roles in modulating proteostasis in tumors. *Cells*, *8*(1), 4.
Egel, R. (2012). Life's order, complexity, organization, and its thermodynamic–holistic imperatives. *Life*, *2*(4), 323–363.

Espinosa-Diez, C., Miguel, V., Mennerich, D., Kietzmann, T., Sánchez-Pérez, P., Cadenas, S., & Lamas, S. (2015). Antioxidant responses and cellular adjustments to oxidative stress. *Redox Biology*, *6*, 183–197.

Evans, C. G., Chang, L., & Gestwicki, J. E. (2010). Heat shock protein 70 (hsp70) as an emerging drug target. *Journal of Medicinal Chemistry*, *53*(12), 4585–4602.

Fares, M. A. (2014). The evolution of protein moonlighting: Adaptive traps and promiscuity in the chaperonins. *Biochemical Society Transactions*, *42*(6), 1709.

Foster, K. R., & Bell, T. (2012). Competition, not cooperation, dominates interactions among culturable microbial species. *Current Biology*, *22*(19), 1845–1850.

Fujimoto, M., & Nakai, A. (2010). The heat shock factor family and adaptation to proteotoxic stress. *The FEBS Journal*, *277*(20), 4112–4125.

Fulda, S., Gorman, A. M., Hori, O., & Samali, A. (2010). Cellular stress responses: Cell survival and cell death. *International Journal of Cell Biology*, *2010*.

Garbett, N. C., & Chaires, J. B. (2012). Thermodynamic studies for drug design and screening. *Expert Opinion on Drug Discovery*, 7(4), 299–314.

Genereux, J. C., & Wiseman, R. L. (2015). Regulating extracellular proteostasis capacity through the unfolded protein response. *Prion*, *9*(1), 10–21.

Ghasemi, M., Jelodar, N. B., Modarresi, M., & Bagheri, N. (2013). Morphological response of German chamomile to heat stress accompanies salicylic acid-mediated under field conditions. *International Journal of Agriculture and Crop Sciences*, *5*(7), 756.

Gilbert, S. F., Bosch, T. C., & Ledón-Rettig, C. (2015). Eco-Evo-Devo: Developmental symbiosis and developmental plasticity as evolutionary agents. *Nature Reviews Genetics*, *16*(10), 611.

Glansdorff, N., Xu, Y., & Labedan, B. (2008). The last universal common ancestor: Emergence, constitution and genetic legacy of an elusive forerunner. *Biology Direct*, *3*(1), 29.

Goldman, A. W., Burmeister, Y., Cesnulevicius, K., Herbert, M., Kane, M., Lescheid, D., … St Laurent, G. (2015). Bioregulatory systems medicine: An innovative approach to integrating the science of molecular networks, inflammation, and systems biology with the patient's autoregulatory capacity? *Frontiers in Physiology*, *6*, 225.

Gomez-Verjan, J. C., Vazquez-Martinez, E. R., Rivero-Segura, N. A., & Medina-Campos, R. H. (2018). The RNA world of human ageing. *Human Genetics*, *137*(11–12), 865–879.

Gorenberg, E. L., & Chandra, S. S. (2017). The role of co-chaperones in synaptic proteostasis and neurodegenerative disease. *Frontiers in Neuroscience*, *11*, 248.

Gorgoulis, V. G., Pefani, D. E., Pateras, I. S., & Trougakos, I. P. (2018). Integrating the DNA damage and protein stress responses during cancer development and treatment. *The Journal of Pathology*, *246*(1), 12–40.

Hauryliuk, V., Atkinson, G. C., Murakami, K. S., Tenson, T., & Gerdes, K. (2015). Recent functional insights into the role of (p) ppGpp in bacterial physiology. *Nature Reviews Microbiology*, *13*(5), 298.

Hill, C. B., Czauderna, T., Klapperstück, M., Roessner, U., & Schreiber, F. (2015). Metabolomics, standards, and metabolic modeling for synthetic biology in plants. *Frontiers in Bioengineering and Biotechnology*, *3*, 167.

Hipp, M. S., Kasturi, P., & Hartl, F. U. (2019). The proteostasis network and its decline in ageing. *Nature Reviews Molecular Cell Biology*, *1*.

Hoelzer, G. A., Smith, E., & Pepper, J. W. (2006). On the logical relationship between natural selection and self-organization. *Journal of Evolutionary Biology*, *19*(6), 1785–1794.

Hoenigsberg, H. (2003). Evolution without speciation but with selection: LUCA, the last universal common ancestor in Gilbert's RNA world. *Genetics and Molecular Research*, *2*(4), 366–375.

Hordijk, W. (2016). Evolution of autocatalytic sets in computational models of chemical reaction networks. *Origins of Life and Evolution of Biospheres*, *46*(2–3), 233–245.

Hordijk, W., & Steel, M. (2017). Chasing the tail: The emergence of autocatalytic networks. *Biosystems*, *152*, 1–10.

Hordijk, W., & Steel, M. (2018). Autocatalytic networks at the basis of life's origin and organization. *Life*, *8*(4), 62.
Horowitz, M. (2015). Epigenetics and cytoprotection with heat acclimation. *Journal of Applied Physiology*, *120*(6), 702–710.
Hurst, G. D. (2017). Extended genomes: Symbiosis and evolution. *Interface Focus*, 7(5), 20170001.
Ikwegbue, P., Masamba, P., Oyinloye, B., & Kappo, A. (2018). Roles of heat shock proteins in apoptosis, oxidative stress, human inflammatory diseases, and cancer. *Pharmaceuticals*, *11*(1), 2.
Ildefonso, M. (2015). Elements of the cellular metabolic structure. *Frontiers in Molecular Biosciences*, *2*.
Ito, K., & Suda, T. (2014). Metabolic requirements for the maintenance of self-renewing stem cells. *Nature Reviews Molecular Cell Biology*, *15*(4), 243.
Ivanitskii, G. R. (2017). Self-organizing dynamic stability of far-from-equilibrium biological systems. *Physics-Uspekhi*, *60*(7), 705.
Jarosz, D. F., & Lindquist, S. (2010). Hsp90 and environmental stress transform the adaptive value of natural genetic variation. *Science*, *330*(6012), 1820–1824.
Jha, S. K., & Udgaonkar, J. B. (2010). Free energy barriers in protein folding and unfolding reactions. *Current Science*, *99*(4), 457–475.
Jovel, J., Dieleman, L. A., Kao, D., Mason, A. L., & Wine, E. (2018). *The human gut microbiome in health and disease*. In *Metagenomics*. Academic Press. (pp. 197–213).
Kaneko, K., & Furusawa, C. (2018). Macroscopic theory for evolving biological systems akin to thermodynamics. *Annual Review of Biophysics*, *47*, 273–290.
Kirchhoff, M. D., & Froese, T. (2017). Where there is life there is mind: In support of a strong life-mind continuity thesis. *Entropy*, *19*(4), 169.
Klaips, C. L., Jayaraj, G. G., & Hartl, F. U. (2018). Pathways of cellular proteostasis in aging and disease. *The Journal of Cell Biology*, *217*(1), 51–63.
Kotas, M. E., & Medzhitov, R. (2015). Homeostasis, inflammation, and disease susceptibility. *Cell*, *160*(5), 816–827.
Kurakin, A. (2011). The self-organizing fractal theory as a universal discovery method: The phenomenon of life. *Theoretical Biology and Medical Modelling*, *8*(1), 4.
Kurutas, E. B. (2015). The importance of antioxidants which play the role in cellular response against oxidative/nitrosative stress: Current state. *Nutrition Journal*, *15*(1), 71.
Labbadia, J., & Morimoto, R. I. (2015). The biology of proteostasis in aging and disease. *Annual Review of Biochemistry*, *84*, 435–464.
Lachnit, T., Bosch, T. C., & Deines, P. (2019). Exposure of the host-associated microbiome to nutrient-rich conditions may lead to dysbiosis and disease development—An evolutionary perspective. *MBio*, *10*(3), e00355-19.
Lancet, D., Zidovetzki, R., & Markovitch, O. (2018). Systems protobiology: Origin of life in lipid catalytic networks. *Journal of the Royal Society Interface*, *15*(144), 20180159.
Latorre, V., Mattenberger, F., & Geller, R. (2018). Chaperoning the mononegavirales: Current knowledge and future directions. *Viruses*, *10*(12), 699.
Lee, H.Y., Chao, J. C., Cheng, K.Y., & Leu, J.Y. (2018). Misfolding-prone proteins are reversibly sequestered to an Hsp42-associated granule upon chronological aging. *Journal of Cell Science*, *131*(16), jcs220202.
Lefevre, J. G., Chiu, H. S., Combes, A. N., Vanslambrouck, J. M., Ju, A., Hamilton, N. A., & Little, M. H. (2017). Self-organisation after embryonic kidney dissociation is driven via selective adhesion of ureteric epithelial cells. *Development*, *144*(6), 1087–1096.
Letelier, J. C., Marın, G., & Mpodozis, J. (2003). Autopoietic and (M, R) systems. *Journal of Theoretical Biology*, *222*(2), 261–272.
Lindquist, S. L., & Kelly, J. W. (2011). Chemical and biological approaches for adapting proteostasis to ameliorate protein misfolding and aggregation diseases—Progress and prognosis. *Cold Spring Harbor Perspectives in Biology*, *3*(12), a004507.

Liu, M., Li, X., Liu, Y., & Cao, B. (2013). Regulation of flavanone 3-hydroxylase gene involved in the flavonoid biosynthesis pathway in response to UV-B radiation and drought stress in the desert plant, Reaumuria soongorica. *Plant Physiology and Biochemistry*, *73*, 161–167.

Lucia, U. (2015). Bioengineering thermodynamics of biological cells. *Theoretical Biology and Medical Modelling*, *12*(1), 29.

Lupoli, T. J., Vaubourgeix, J., Burns-Huang, K., & Gold, B. (2018). Targeting the proteostasis network for mycobacterial drug discovery. *ACS Infectious Diseases*, *4*(4), 478–498.

MacIver, N. J., Michalek, R. D., & Rathmell, J. C. (2013). Metabolic regulation ofT lymphocytes. *Annual Review of Immunology*, *31*, 259–283.

Maguire, M., & Maguire, G. (2019). Gut dysbiosis, leaky gut, and intestinal epithelial proliferation in neurological disorders: Towards the development of a new therapeutic using amino acids, prebiotics, probiotics, and postbiotics. *Reviews in the Neurosciences*, *30*(2), 179–201.

Maiuri, L., Raia, V., & Kroemer, G. (2017). Strategies for the etiological therapy of cystic fibrosis. *Cell Death and Differentiation*, *24*(11), 1825.

Maleki, F., Afra Khosravi, A. N., Taghinejad, H., & Azizian, M. (2016). Bacterial heat shock protein activity. *Journal of Clinical and Diagnostic Research: JCDR*, *10*(3), BE01.

Mao, L., & Franke, J. (2013). Hormesis in aging and neurodegeneration—A prodigy awaiting dissection. *International Journal of Molecular Sciences*, *14*(7), 13109–13128.

Mao, L., & Franke, J. (2015). Symbiosis, dysbiosis, and rebiosis—The value of metaproteomics in human microbiome monitoring. *Proteomics*, *15*(5–6), 1142–1151.

Mardones, P., Martínez, G., & Hetz, C. (2015). Control of systemic proteostasis by the nervous system. *Trends in Cell Biology*, *25*(1), 1–10.

Maresca, B., & Schwartz, J. H. (2006). Sudden origins: A general mechanism of evolution based on stress protein concentration and rapid environmental change. *Anatomical Record Part B, New Anatomist*, *289*(1), 38–46.

Marijuán, P. C., Navarro, J., & del Moral, R. (2010). On prokaryotic intelligence: Strategies for sensing the environment. *Biosystems*, *99*(2), 94–103.

Marijuán, P. C., Navarro, J., & del Moral, R. (2015). How the living is in the world: An inquiry into the informational choreographies of life. *Progress in Biophysics and Molecular Biology*, *119*(3), 469–480.

Matsuno, K. (2017). From quantum measurement to biology via retrocausality. *Progress in Biophysics and Molecular Biology*, *131*, 131–140.

Mercado, G., & Hetz, C. (2017). Drug repurposing to target proteostasis and prevent neurodegeneration: Accelerating translational efforts. *Brain*, *140*(6), 1544–1547.

Metallo, C. M., & Vander Heiden, M. G. (2013). Understanding metabolic regulation and its influence on cell physiology. *Molecular Cell*, *49*(3), 388–398.

Migicovsky, Z., Yao, Y., & Kovalchuk, I. (2014). Transgenerational phenotypic and epigenetic changes in response to heat stress in *Arabidopsis thaliana*. *Plant Signaling & Behavior*, *9*(2), e27971.

Miller, W. (2016). Cognition, information fields and hologenomic entanglement: Evolution in light and shadow. *Biology*, *5*(2), 21.

Moradali, M. F., Ghods, S., & Rehm, B. H. (2017). Pseudomonas aeruginosa lifestyle: A paradigm for adaptation, survival, and persistence. *Frontiers in Cellular and Infection Microbiology*, *7*, 39.

Moral, R. D., González, M., Navarro, J., & Marijuán, P. C. (2011). From genomics to scientomics: Expanding the bioinformation paradigm. *Information*, *2*(4), 651–671.

Morano, K. A., Grant, C. M., & Moye-Rowley, W. S. (2012). The response to heat shock and oxidative stress in *Saccharomyces cerevisiae*. *Genetics*, *190*(4), 1157–1195.

Moreno, A. (2016). Some conceptual issues in the transition from chemistry to biology. *History and Philosophy of the Life Sciences*, *38*(4), 16.

Muraille, E. (2018). Diversity generator mechanisms are essential components of biological systems: The two queen hypothesis. *Frontiers in Microbiology*, *9*, 223.

Na, D., Kim, T. Y., & Lee, S. Y. (2010). Construction and optimization of synthetic pathways in metabolic engineering. *Current Opinion in Microbiology*, *13*(3), 363–370.

Nousala, S. (2012). Emerging "living" communities-scalability of knowledge transfer in complex systems. *Constraints*, *12*, 14.

O'Malley, M. A. (2015). Endosymbiosis and its implications for evolutionary theory. *Proceedings of the National Academy of Sciences*, *112*(33), 10270–10277.

Pan, T. (2013). Adaptive translation as a mechanism of stress response and adaptation. *Annual Review of Genetics*, *47*, 121–137.

Park, C. J., & Seo, Y. S. (2015). Heat shock proteins: A review of the molecular chaperones for plant immunity. *Plant Pathology Journal*, *31*(4), 323.

Pita, L., Rix, L., Slaby, B. M., Franke, A., & Hentschel, U. (2018). The sponge holobiont in a changing ocean: From microbes to ecosystems. *Microbiome*, *6*(1), 46.

Plasson, R., Brandenburg, A., Jullien, L., & Bersini, H. (2011). Autocatalysis: At the root of self-replication. *Artificial Life*, *17*(3), 219–236.

Porporato, P. E., Filigheddu, N., Bravo-San Pedro, J. M., Kroemer, G., & Galluzzi, L. (2018). Mitochondrial metabolism and cancer. *Cell Research*, *28*(3), 265.

Powers, E. T., & Balch, W. E. (2013). Diversity in the origins of proteostasis networks—A driver for protein function in evolution. *Nature Reviews Molecular Cell Biology*, *14*(4), 237.

Powers, E. T., Morimoto, R. I., Dillin, A., Kelly, J. W., & Balch, W. E. (2009). Biological and chemical approaches to diseases of proteostasis deficiency. *Annual Review of Biochemistry*, *78*, 959–991.

Pröschel, M., Detsch, R., Boccaccini, A. R., & Sonnewald, U. (2015). Engineering of metabolic pathways by artificial enzyme channels. *Frontiers in Bioengineering and Biotechnology*, *3*, 168.

Qu, A. L., Ding, Y. F., Jiang, Q., & Zhu, C. (2013). Molecular mechanisms of the plant heat stress response. *Biochemical and Biophysical Research Communications*, *432*(2), 203–207.

Ramakrishnan, R., Houben, B., Rousseau, F., & Schymkowitz, J. (2019). Differential proteostatic regulation of insoluble and abundant proteins. *Bioinformatics (Oxford, England)*, pii: btz214.

Recordati, G., & Bellini, T. G. (2004). A definition of internal constancy and homeostasis in the context of non-equilibrium thermodynamics. *Experimental Physiology*, *89*(1), 27–38.

Rickard, A. H., Palmer, R. J., Jr., Blehert, D. S., Campagna, S. R., Semmelhack, M. F., Egland, P. G., ... Kolenbrander, P. E. (2006). Autoinducer 2: A concentration-dependent signal for mutualistic bacterial biofilm growth. *Molecular Microbiology*, *60*(6), 1446–1456.

Root-Bernstein, R. S., & Dillon, P. F. (1997). Molecular complementarity I: The complementarity theory of the origin and evolution of life. *Journal of Theoretical Biology*, *188*(4), 447–479.

Round, J. L., & Mazmanian, S. K. (2009). The gut microbiota shapes intestinal immune responses during health and disease. *Nature Reviews Immunology*, *9*(5), 313.

Saad, N. Y. (2018). A ribonucleopeptide world at the origin of life. *Journal of Systematics and Evolution*, *56*(1), 1–13.

Saetzler, K., Sonnenschein, C., & Soto, A. M. (2011). Systems biology beyond networks: Generating order from disorder through self-organization. *Seminars in Cancer Biology*, *21*(3), 165. NIH Public Access.

Saibil, H. (2013). Chaperone machines for protein folding, unfolding and disaggregation. *Nature Reviews Molecular Cell Biology*, *14*(10), 630.

Scirè, A., & Annovazzi-Lodi, V. (2017). Self-organization in a diversity induced thermodynamics. *PLoS One*, *12*(12), e0188753.

Seeley, T. D. (2002). When is self-organization used in biological systems? *The Biological Bulletin*, *202*(3), 314–318.

Shalgi, R., Hurt, J. A., Lindquist, S., & Burge, C. B. (2014). Widespread inhibition of posttranscriptional splicing shapes the cellular transcriptome following heat shock. *Cell Reports*, 7(5), 1362–1370.

Silverman, M. N., & Deuster, P. A. (2014). Biological mechanisms underlying the role of physical fitness in health and resilience. *Interface Focus*, *4*(5), 20140040.
Soen, Y., Knafo, M., & Elgart, M. (2015). A principle of organization which facilitates broad Lamarckian-like adaptations by improvisation. *Biology Direct*, *10*(1), 68.
Somvanshi, P. R., & Venkatesh, K.V. (2014). A conceptual review on systems biology in health and diseases: From biological networks to modern therapeutics. *Systems and Synthetic Biology*, *8*(1), 99–116.
Stetler, R. A., Gan, Y., Zhang, W., Liou, A. K., Gao, Y., Cao, G., & Chen, J. (2010). Heat shock proteins: Cellular and molecular mechanisms in the central nervous system. *Progress in Neurobiology*, *92*(2), 184–211.
Storey, K. B., & Wu, C. W. (2013). Stress response and adaptation: A new molecular toolkit for the 21st century. *Comparative Biochemistry and Physiology Part A: Molecular & Integrative Physiology*, *165*(4), 417–428.
Swenson, R. (1992). Autocatakinetics, yes—Autopoiesis, no: Steps toward a unified theory of evolutionary ordering. *International Journal of General Systems*, *21*(2), 207–228.
Swenson, R. (1997). Autocatakinetics, evolution, and the law of maximum entropy production: A principled foundation towards the study of human ecology. *Advances in Human Ecology*, *6*, 1–48.
Swenson, R. (1998). *Spontaneous order, evolution, and autocatakinetics: The nomological basis for the emergence of meaning*. In *Evolutionary systems*. Dordrecht: Springer. (pp. 155–180).
Takeuchi, T., Suzuki, M., Fujikake, N., Popiel, H. A., Kikuchi, H., Futaki, S., ... Nagai, Y. (2015). Intercellular chaperone transmission via exosomes contributes to maintenance of protein homeostasis at the organismal level. *Proceedings of the National Academy of Sciences*, *112*(19), E2497–E2506.
Torday, J. (2015). Homeostasis as the mechanism of evolution. *Biology*, *4*(3), 573–590.
Torday, J. (2016). The emergence of physiology and form: Natural selection revisited. *Biology*, *5*(2), 15.
Triandafillou, C. G., Katanski, C. D., Dinner, A. R., & Drummond, D. A. (2018). *Transient intracellular acidification regulates the core transcriptional heat shock response*. . Available at SSRN 3276046.
Vabulas, R. M., Raychaudhuri, S., Hayer-Hartl, M., & Hartl, F. U. (2010). Protein folding in the cytoplasm and the heat shock response. *Cold Spring Harbor Perspectives in Biology*, *2*(12), a004390.
Vallino, J. J. (2010). Ecosystem biogeochemistry considered as a distributed metabolic network ordered by maximum entropy production. *Philosophical Transactions of the Royal Society, B: Biological Sciences*, *365*(1545), 1417–1427.
van Oosten-Hawle, P., & Morimoto, R. I. (2014). Organismal proteostasis: Role of cell-nonautonomous regulation and transcellular chaperone signaling. *Genes & Development*, *28*(14), 1533–1543.
van Oosten-Hawle, P., Porter, R. S., & Morimoto, R. I. (2013). Regulation of organismal proteostasis by transcellular chaperone signaling. *Cell*, *153*(6), 1366–1378.
Verghese, J., Abrams, J., Wang, Y., & Morano, K. A. (2012). Biology of the heat shock response and protein chaperones: Budding yeast (*Saccharomyces cerevisiae*) as a model system. *Microbiology and Molecular Biology Reviews*, *76*(2), 115–158.
Vijver, G., Salthe, S. N., & Delpos, M. (Eds.), (2013). *Evolutionary systems: Biological and epistemological perspectives on selection and self-organization*. Heidelberg: Springer Science & Business Media.
Vitreschak, A. G., Rodionov, D. A., Mironov, A. A., & Gelfand, M. S. (2004). Riboswitches: The oldest mechanism for the regulation of gene expression? *Trends in Genetics*, *20*(1), 44–50.
Wahid, A., Gelani, S., Ashraf, M., & Foolad, M. R. (2007). Heat tolerance in plants: An overview. *Environmental and Experimental Botany*, *61*(3), 199–223.

Wang, W., Vinocur, B., Shoseyov, O., & Altman, A. (2004). Role of plant heat-shock proteins and molecular chaperones in the abiotic stress response. *Trends in Plant Science*, *9*(5), 244–252.

Webster, N. S., & Thomas, T. (2016). The sponge hologenome. *MBio*, 7(2), e00135-16.

Wei, Y., & Murphy, E. R. (2016). Temperature-dependent regulation of bacterial gene expression by RNA thermometers. In M. L. Larramendy & S. Solonesky (Eds.), *Nucleic acids-from basic aspects to laboratory tools* (pp. 157–181). London: IntechOpen.

Wei, G., Xi, W., Nussinov, R., & Ma, B. (2016). Protein ensembles: How does nature harness thermodynamic fluctuations for life? The diverse functional roles of conformational ensembles in the cell. *Chemical Reviews*, *116*(11), 6516–6551.

West, C. E., Jenmalm, M. C., & Prescott, S. L. (2015). The gut microbiota and its role in the development of allergic disease: A wider perspective. *Clinical & Experimental Allergy*, *45*(1), 43–53.

West, J. D., Wang, Y., & Morano, K. A. (2012). Small molecule activators of the heat shock response: Chemical properties, molecular targets, and therapeutic promise. *Chemical Research in Toxicology*, *25*(10), 2036–2053.

Wolynes, P. G. (2015). Evolution, energy landscapes and the paradoxes of protein folding. *Biochimie*, *119*, 218–230.

Wosniack, M. E., da Luz, M. G. E., & Schulman, L. S. (2017). Punctuated equilibrium as an emergent process and its modified thermodynamic characterization. *Journal of Theoretical Biology*, *412*, 113–122.

Yang, Y., & Sauve, A. A. (2016). NAD+ metabolism: Bioenergetics, signaling and manipulation for therapy. *Biochimica et Biophysica Acta (BBA)—Proteins and Proteomics*, *1864*(12), 1787–1800.

Yarus, M. (2011). Getting past the RNA world: The initial Darwinian ancestor. *Cold Spring Harbor Perspectives in Biology*, *3*(4), a003590.

Yerbury, J. J., Ooi, L., Dillin, A., Saunders, D. N., Hatters, D. M., Beart, P. M., … Ecroyd, H. (2016). Walking the tightrope: Proteostasis and neurodegenerative disease. *Journal of Neurochemistry*, *137*(4), 489–505.

Yufik, Y. M. (2019). The understanding capacity and information dynamics in the human brain. *Entropy*, *21*(3), 308.

Zimmermann, A., Bauer, M. A., Kroemer, G., Madeo, F., & Carmona-Gutierrez, D. (2014). When less is more: Hormesis against stress and disease. *Microbial Cell*, *1*(5), 150.

Zorov, D. B., Juhaszova, M., & Sollott, S. J. (2014). Mitochondrial reactive oxygen species (ROS) and ROS-induced ROS release. *Physiological Reviews*, *94*(3), 909–950.

Zuo, D., Subjeck, J., & Wang, X. Y. (2016). Unfolding the role of large heat shock proteins: New insights and therapeutic implications. *Frontiers in Immunology*, 7, 75.

CHAPTER 10

Biophysics applications in drug discovery: Working toward a new integrative model

A poet once said, 'The whole universe is in a glass of wine.' We will probably never know in what sense he meant it, for poets do not write to be understood. But it is true that if we look at a glass of wine closely enough we see the entire universe. There are the things of physics: the twisting liquid which evaporates depending on the wind and weather, the reflection in the glass; and our imagination adds atoms. The glass is a distillation of the earth's rocks, and in its composition we see the secrets of the universe's age, and the evolution of stars. What strange array of chemicals are in the wine? How did they come to be? There are the ferments, the enzymes, the substrates, and the products. There in wine is found the great generalization; all life is fermentation. Nobody can discover the chemistry of wine without discovering, as did Louis Pasteur, the cause of much disease. How vivid is the claret, pressing its existence into the consciousness that watches it! If our small minds, for some convenience, divide this glass of wine, this universe, into parts -- physics, biology, geology, astronomy, psychology, and so on -- remember that nature does not know it! So let us put it all back together, not forgetting ultimately what it is for. Let it give us one more final pleasure; drink it and forget it all!

Richard P. Feynman (1918–88)

10.1 Introduction

Biophysical methods are the platform for evaluating the impact of new drugs in which evolutionary models can be combined with the mechanisms of action in the design of promising molecules (Holdgate et al., 2013; Renaud et al., 2016). Thus, drug screening platforms based on biophysical methods allow us to obtain information about the actions of drugs in metabolic networks, as well as the metabolomic changes that the

Molecular Evolutionary Models in Drug Discovery
https://doi.org/10.1016/B978-0-12-817613-9.00010-9

patient presents (human holobiont) as the treatment progresses (Docci, Parrott, Krähenbühl, & Fowler, 2019; Dorrestein, Mazmanian, & Knight, 2014; Kell, 2013). It is also possible to integrate the functionality and the therapeutic targets, as well as their effects on the adaptive responses of the host, with which we can enter an era of personalized pharmacology (Fig. 1) (Docci et al., 2019; Dorrestein et al., 2014; Kell, 2013). In this way, a pharmacology system requires a model that evaluates the functionality in correlation with the therapeutic target, as well as with the solubility and cellular permeability, in order to decrease the failure rate in the process and increase the impact on pharmaceutical innovation (Hoelder, Clarke, & Workman, 2012; Trosset & Carbonell, 2015; Wen, Jung, & Li, 2015). Thus the pharmacology of systems to integrate biophysical methods can transcend a new vision of phenotypic assays where the functionality of the therapeutic target in the biological system is the source of information (Hasson & Inglese, 2013; Nussinov, Jang, Tsai, & Cheng, 2019).

In this way, measuring both the absorption and coupling of the drug to the target protein, as well as observing the phenotypic adaptations of the biological system in the same bioassay model, is one of the possibilities that should be considered to develop a robust, reproducible, and automatable screening platform (Joslin et al., 2018; Möller & Slack, 2010; Saltepe, Kehribar, Su Yirmibeşoğlu, & Şafak Şeker, 2017). Thus, a modern biophysical drug discovery platform must be able to determine the coevolution, interactions, and symbiosis present in a holobiontic system, in order to give a model of personalized medicine and increase the prediction of clinical response (Fig. 2) (Jain, 2013; Mirsadeghi & Larijani, 2017; Stern,

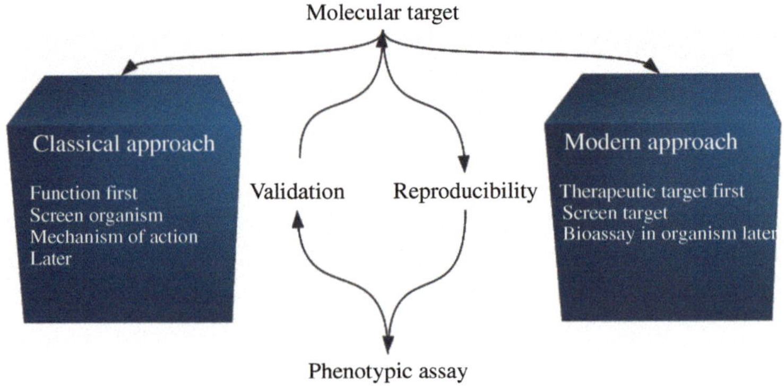

Fig. 1 Screening models in drug discovery.

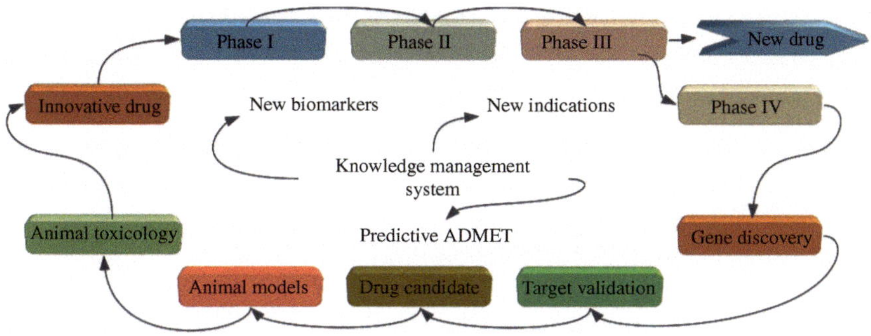

Fig. 2 Drug discovery process based on systems pharmacology.

Schurdak, Bahar, Berg, & Taylor, 2016). In this search for novel screening platforms in an integrative model it is necessary to include synthetic biology as a biomimetic approach in which, in a multi-trans-inter disciplinary approach, it is possible to determine the cognition of the biological system by allowing knowledge, and modify the metabolic and signaling networks that are part of the evolutionary phenomenon (Renda, Hammerling, & Barrick, 2014; Smith, van Sluijs, & Fleck, 2017; Stano, 2019).

Likewise, designing and implementing biomimetic models of biological systems will allow us to observe the metabolic pathways that drive self-organization and the autopoietic response, with which it will be possible to determine and evaluate new therapeutic targets (Mori & Shirai, 2018; Nikolaev, 2010; Schmidt-Dannert & Lopez-Gallego, 2016). Additionally, the possibility of making epigenetic and mutational modifications of the biosynthetic pathways that regulate the adaptive response will be able to promote the biotechnological development of a great variety of secondary metabolites, as well as to study the capacity of optimization and the biological function on the primary metabolism that these possess (Gacek & Strauss, 2012; Guerriero et al., 2018; Kumar & Prasad, 2011; Pickens, Tang, & Chooi, 2011). Likewise, the use of cellular adaptive machinery for the development of new products is a promising field in biotechnology in order to have more and better chemically diverse compounds in a green chemistry model (Hallmann, 2015; Le Feuvre & Scrutton, 2018; Singh & Pelaez, 2008; Smanski et al., 2016). Therefore, the objective of this chapter is to carry out an integrative analysis of evolutionary models in combination with biophysical methods for the design and implementation of a rational strategy for the discovery of new medicines (Madani Tonekaboni, Soltan Ghoraie, Manem, & Haibe-Kains, 2016; Ramsay, Popovic-Nikolic, Nikolic, Uliassi, & Bolognesi, 2018).

10.2 Systems biology in an evolutionary model in drug discovery

The evolution in the biology of systems prevents all reductionism and is also useful in the discovery of new drugs, their combinations, as well as their optimization. All this is done by driving the action of a drug as a system and not as a specific action on a given therapeutic target (Fig. 3) (Al-Ali, 2016; Danhof, 2016; Sánchez-Rodríguez et al., 2017; Zou, Zheng, Li, & Su, 2013). Therefore, this type of approach requires a multifactorial analysis of the biological modifications induced by the mechanism of pharmacological action in which the genomic, proteomic, epigenomic, metabolomics, and interactomic parameters are correlated in a multiomics study platform (Liang & Kelemen, 2017; Rai, Saito, & Yamazaki, 2017; Shi-Kai et al., 2015; Tebani & Bekri, 2019). But it is important to take this comprehensive analysis to study the dynamics of the biological system over time, as well as its thermodynamic equilibrium in the ability to share the entropy with other individuals (Haddad, 2017; Ouldridge, 2018; Selvarajoo, 2015).

Likewise, within the biological system under pharmacological effects enthalpy should be determined (amount of energy that the system exchanges with the environment) as a measure of optimization of drug design to obtain adequate ADMET properties (absorption, distribution, metabolism, excretion and toxicology) (Claveria-Gimeno, Vega, Abian, &

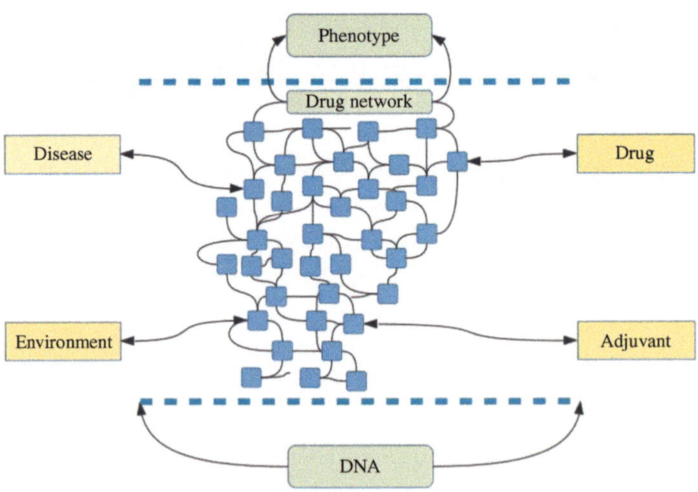

Fig. 3 Pharmacology of systems in complex biological systems.

Velazquez-Campoy, 2017; Geschwindner, Ulander, & Johansson, 2015; Yang et al., 2018). This enthalpy determines the pharmacological action of the drug and the capacity of the biological system in treatment to establish metabolic and communication networks as an adaptive response to the present chemical modulation (Derbal, 2018; Egorova, Gordeev, & Ananikov, 2017; Ma & Zhao, 2014). Likewise, thermodynamic properties determine the permeability properties of innovative formulations that optimize absorption and activity, such as the antimicrobial activity of ionic liquids (ILs), capable of penetrating biofilms with effectivity (Aditya et al., 2018; Benedetto & Ballone, 2018; Zakrewsky et al., 2014). Thus, in the application of thermodynamics in drug discovery, biophysical methods capable of measuring and analyzing multiparameter data are necessary, such as surface plasmon resonance (SPR), isothermal titration calorimetry (ITC), nuclear magnetic resonance (NMR), and mass spectrometry (MS). With these, it is possible to determine the adaptive modifications of the biological system as the treatment proceeds and the clinical outcome can be predicted (Amaro et al., 2018; Gohlke et al., 2018; Ingber, 2018; Shimada et al., 2018).

10.3 Biophysical methods and thermodynamic drug discovery

The flow of energy and the sharing of entropy in a self-organized system make up the metabolic and communication networks of open biological systems, which determine homeostasis and fitness (Ildefonso, 2015; Sengupta, Stemmler, & Friston, 2013; Zivieri, Pacini, Finocchio, & Carpentieri, 2017). Thus, a program of design and development of new drugs should aim to determine the pharmacological activity in the metabolic functionality of the system, in order to establish the dynamics of multienzyme processes that are the therapeutic targets in medicinal chemistry (Borhani & Shaw, 2012; Chubukov, Mukhopadhyay, Petzold, Keasling, & Martín, 2016; Vangala et al., 2011). Likewise, the concept of ligand and receptor should be transcended in order to arrive at the notion of adaptive molecular networks, which, when modified in the search for equilibrium, need to be evaluated in their capacity to optimize the energy flows of the system as well as their autonomy (Doerr, Harvey, Noé, & De Fabritiis, 2016; Farnsworth, 2018; Juster, Russell, Almeida, & Picard, 2016).

In this way, the application of biophysical techniques in the process of drug screening can give a comprehensive view of the pharmacological activity on open biological systems (Camacho, Collins, Powers, Costello, & Collins, 2018; Martinez Molina & Nordlund, 2016; Schuetz et al., 2017). Such is the case of NMR-based metabolomics, which can obtain data on the biochemistry of an organism at different moments of its interaction, symbiosis, and evolution, becoming a multiparametric evaluation of an open self-organized biological system (Gogna, Sharma, Gupta, Dorai, & Prasad, 2017; Markley et al., 2017; Pimenta, Kim, Verpoorte, & Choi, 2013). This method also allows us to evaluate the evolution of the metabolome and to elucidate the adaptive metabolic pathways used in response to environmental and pharmacological agents (Johnson, Ivanisevic, & Siuzdak, 2016; Peng, Li, & Peng, 2015; Prosser, Larrouy-Maumus, & de Carvalho, 2014). Additionally, the possibility of establishing metabolic pathways and fluxomics (metabolic reactions within the system), as well as the chemometrics of interacting species, will be an important factor to apply this type of method in the study of homeostasis inside the holobiont (Fig. 4) (Brucker & Bordenstein, 2012; Chaston & Douglas, 2012; Rosato et al., 2018).

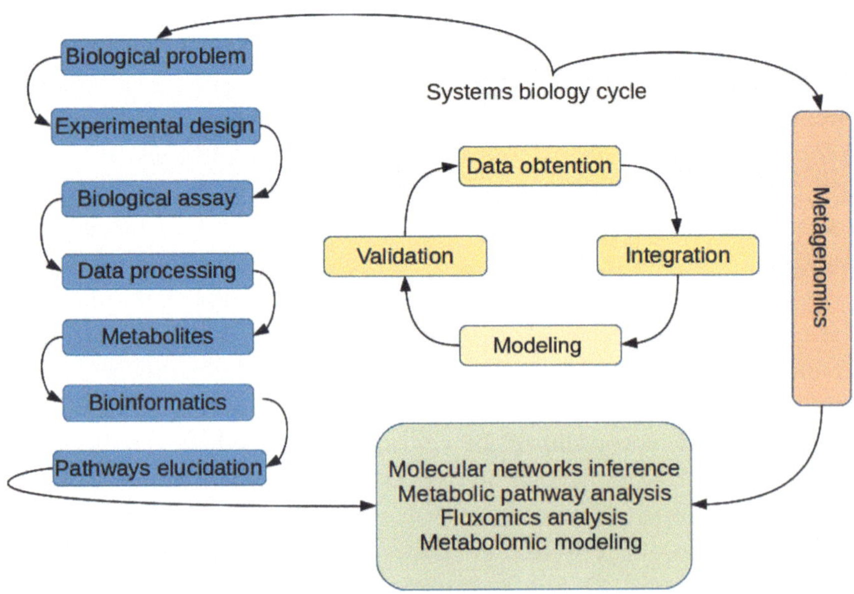

Fig. 4 Metabolomic modeling of biological systems.

10.4 The metabolomics of homeostasis

The observation of the biological model in equilibrium during the pharmacological action allows us to determine how it adapts to maintain homeostasis through epigenetic regulatory processes and the hormetic response (Calabrese, Cornelius, Dinkova-Kostova, Calabrese, & Mattson, 2010; Cortese-Krott et al., 2017; Vaiserman, 2011). In this way, evaluating the metabolomic biomarkers that determine the homeostasis in the biological system, as well as the symbiotic relationships that allow the flow of energy in the metabolic networks, will allow obtaining important information of the pharmacological action process in the cure of diverse diseases (Klassen et al., 2017; Metallo & Vander Heiden, 2013; Vernocchi et al., 2012; Wishart, 2016). Likewise, the physiology of the biological system under different adaptive conditions against oxidative stress may be determined, in order to develop novel drugs that promote the coevolution of the holobiont (Rosenberg & Zilber-Rosenberg, 2018; Scott et al., 2017; Thomas et al., 2017). In addition, the analysis of the hormetic response to xenobiotics can be compared to determine from the evaluation of the pharmacological activity the possibility of toxicity and adverse reactions from an integrative model of the in vitro biological test (Boncler et al., 2017; Hartung et al., 2017; Miller, Prince, Mouch, & Boyd, 2019; Tóth, Brózik, Szakács, Sarkadi, & Hegedüs, 2015).

Thus, a biological model that can predict the modifications of the hologenome under the different therapeutic molecules and that also promotes the restoration of symbiotic interactions within the holobiont must use the pharmacology of systems to establish the metabolomic profile of the biomarkers involved in each disruption known metabolic syndrome that results in disease (Postler & Ghosh, 2017; Rooks & Garrett, 2016; Selber-Hnatiw et al., 2017; Sharma, Jaiswal, Chaudhary, & Sharma, 2017). Then, in a model of the therapy, the functionality to reach the balance of the biological system will be required to integrate the metabolomics of the populations of biological individuals in constant interaction within the holobiont to enter the design and development of symbiotic drugs that configure a personalized evolutionary medicine (Andraos et al., 2019; Coleman et al., 2018; Koskella, Hall, & Metcalf, 2017; Rook, Bäckhed, Levin, McFall-Ngai, & McLean, 2017).

10.5 Metagenomics, metabolomics, and symbiotic drugs

The data obtained by means of metagenomic methods regarding the biological species involved in the symbiosis in conjunction with the metabolomics of the interactions offers us a perspective of the patient as a holobiont whose metabolic networks are in disruption (Cui et al., 2018; Milani et al., 2017; Preidis & Hotez, 2015; Turnbaugh & Gordon, 2008). This is how it is possible to correlate the biomarkers of the disease with the different microbial populations inside the host, as well as to analyze the changes of the hologenome during the healing process (Antunes, Davies, & Finlay, 2011; Rosenberg & Zilber-Rosenberg, 2011, 2018; Zhao et al., 2012). In this order of ideas, the design and development of symbiotic drugs capable of restoring and maintaining the biological populations belonging to the holobiont, as well as of restoring the metabolic networks that make up the symbiosis, become a necessity for the treatment of chronic diseases, infections and cancer (Mao & Franke, 2015; Porcar, 2019; Shapira, 2016; Shapiro, 2017). In this way, the union between metabolomics and metagenomics is a fundamental piece in the clinical evaluation of this kind of drugs, with the purpose of analyzing the fluctuations in the biomarkers of homeostasis of the patient that allow us to show the result of the clinical outcome (Cronin et al., 2018; Johnson et al., 2016; Tolstikov, 2016; Wei et al., 2018). In addition, in this step toward symbiotic drugs we should check the individual evolutionary chemistry of each holobiont, their adaptations, ability to interact, and stress response to stress, because in these aspects are the targets of action for future biotechnological developments (Chagas, de Cassia Pessotti, Caraballo-Rodríguez, & Pupo, 2018; Richier, Furla, Plantivaux, Merle, & Allemand, 2005; Rosenberg & Zilber-Rosenberg, 2019).

10.6 Biophysical methods in biotechnology

The biophysical methods applied for the discovery of new medicines in biotechnology transcend from the fact of allowing the development of biological systems for the obtaining of new products based on adaptive multispecies processes applied in biotechnological models in which it is required to compare multiparameter measurements under diverse conditions (Babadaei et al., 2018; Best & Lindorff-Larsen, 2018; Katz et al., 2018). Thus, the possibility of determining multiple biomarkers of homeostasis of a biological production system within a bioreactor can be fundamental for the future advancement of a biotechnology that uses complex systems as a source of innovation (Marx et al., 2016; Zahrl, Peña, Mattanovich, & Gasser, 2017). Likewise, the possibility of designing models of bioreactors for biotechnology of systems coupled to microfluidics, biosensors, and biochip platforms is only achieved when a large amount of information on the metabolomics of the system can be correlated through the incubation time (Kakaç, Kosoy, Li, & Pramuanjaroenkij, 2010; Saltepe et al., 2017). Thus the chemical evolution associated with the biotechnology of complex systems will reinforce therapeutic innovation in the search for modern medicines that allow us as a species to continue in our continuum of adaptation, transformation and survival (Avise & Ayala, 2007; Maley et al., 2017).

10.7 Conclusions

A new therapeutic approach that uses evolutionary models in order to develop drugs capable of maintaining the homeostasis of the human biological system becomes necessary (Andersson & Tracey, 2012; Basanta & Anderson, 2017; Basanta, Miodownik, & Baum, 2008). The application of the concepts of thermodynamic equilibrium, self-organization, autopoiesis, and holobiont are key to the development of a modern systems pharmacology. Thus the objective of this approach based on complex living systems should be the discovery and development of multifunctional hybrid compounds capable of restoring molecular networks in the human holobiont and help in the adaptive processes for survival. Likewise, the search for this type of medication requires the integral implementation of several fields in evolutionary chemistry, as well as in metabolomics and metagenomics, to be able to evaluate the changes in the biological systems as the treatment progresses. Finally, this approach should lead us to the concept of symbiotic drugs that maintain interactions and communication within the holobiont and allow us to restore the functionality of the biological system.

References

Aditya, A., Chattopadhyay, S., Jha, D., Gautam, H. K., Maiti, S., & Ganguli, M. (2018). Zinc oxide nanoparticles dispersed in ionic liquids show high antimicrobial efficacy to skin-specific bacteria. *ACS Applied Materials & Interfaces*, *10*(18), 15401–15411.

Al-Ali, H. (2016). The evolution of drug discovery: From phenotypes to targets, and back. *Medicinal Chemistry Communications*, 7(5), 788–798.

Amaro, R. E., Baudry, J., Chodera, J., Demir, Ö., McCammon, J. A., Miao, Y., & Smith, J. C. (2018). Ensemble docking in drug discovery. *Biophysical Journal*, *114*(10), 2271–2278.

Andersson, U., & Tracey, K. J. (2012). Reflex principles of immunological homeostasis. *Annual Review of Immunology*, *30*, 313–335.

Andraos, S., Wake, M., Saffery, R., Burgner, D., Kussmann, M., & O'Sullivan, J. (2019). Perspective: Advancing understanding of population nutrient-health relations via metabolomics and precision phenotypes. *Advances in Nutrition (Bethesda, MD)*, pii: nmz045.

Antunes, L. C. M., Davies, J. E., & Finlay, B. B. (2011). Chemical signaling in the gastrointestinal tract. *F1000 Biology Reports*, *3*.

Avise, J. C., & Ayala, F. J. (2007). In the light of evolution I: Adaptation and complex design. *Proceedings of the National Academy of Sciences, 104*(Suppl. 1), 8563–8566.

Babadaei, M. M. N., Moghaddam, M. F., Solhvand, S., Alizadehmollayaghoob, E., Attar, F., Rajabbeigi, E., ... Falahati, M. (2018). Biophysical, bioinformatical, cellular, and molecular investigations on the effects of graphene oxide nanosheets on the hemoglobin structure and lymphocyte cell cytotoxicity. *International Journal of Nanomedicine, 13*, 6871.

Basanta, D., & Anderson, A. R. A. (2017). Homeostasis back and forth: An ecoevolutionary perspective of cancer. *Cold Spring Harbor Perspectives in Medicine*, 7(9).

Basanta, D., Miodownik, M., & Baum, B. (2008). The evolution of robust development and homeostasis in artificial organisms. *PLoS Computational Biology*, *4*(3), e1000030.

Benedetto, A., & Ballone, P. (2018). Room-temperature ionic liquids and biomembranes: Setting the stage for applications in pharmacology, biomedicine, and bionanotechnology. *Langmuir, 34*(33), 9579–9597.

Best, R. B., & Lindorff-Larsen, K. (2018). Editorial overview: Theory and simulation: Interpreting experimental data at the molecular level. *Current Opinion in Structural Biology, 49*, iv.

Boncler, M., Golanski, J., Lukasiak, M., Redzynia, M., Dastych, J., & Watala, C. (2017). A new approach for the assessment of the toxicity of polyphenol-rich compounds with the use of high content screening analysis. *PLoS One, 12*(6), e0180022.

Borhani, D. W., & Shaw, D. E. (2012). The future of molecular dynamics simulations in drug discovery. *Journal of Computer-Aided Molecular Design, 26*(1), 15–26.

Brucker, R. M., & Bordenstein, S. R. (2012). Speciation by symbiosis. *Trends in Ecology & Evolution, 27*(8), 443–451.

Calabrese, V., Cornelius, C., Dinkova-Kostova, A. T., Calabrese, E. J., & Mattson, M. P. (2010). Cellular stress responses, the hormesis paradigm, and vitagenes: Novel targets for therapeutic intervention in neurodegenerative disorders. *Antioxidants & Redox Signaling, 13*(11), 1763–1811.

Camacho, D. M., Collins, K. M., Powers, R. K., Costello, J. C., & Collins, J. J. (2018). Next-generation machine learning for biological networks. *Cell, 173*(7), 1581–1592.

Chagas, F. O., de Cassia Pessotti, R., Caraballo-Rodríguez, A. M., & Pupo, M. T. (2018). Chemical signaling involved in plant–microbe interactions. *Chemical Society Reviews, 47*(5), 1652–1704.

Chaston, J., & Douglas, A. E. (2012). Making the most of "omics" for symbiosis research. *The Biological Bulletin, 223*(1), 21–29.

Chubukov, V., Mukhopadhyay, A., Petzold, C. J., Keasling, J. D., & Martín, H. G. (2016). Synthetic and systems biology for microbial production of commodity chemicals. *npj Systems Biology and Applications, 2*, 16009.

Claveria-Gimeno, R., Vega, S., Abian, O., & Velazquez-Campoy, A. (2017). A look at ligand binding thermodynamics in drug discovery. *Expert Opinion on Drug Discovery, 12*(4), 363–377.

Coleman, M., Elkins, C., Gutting, B., Mongodin, E., Solano-Aguilar, G., & Walls, I. (2018). Microbiota and dose response: Evolving paradigm of health triangle. *Risk Analysis, 38*(10), 2013–2028.

Cortese-Krott, M. M., Koning, A., Kuhnle, G. G., Nagy, P., Bianco, C. L., Pasch, A., ... Olson, K. R. (2017). The reactive species interactome: Evolutionary emergence, biological significance, and opportunities for redox metabolomics and personalized medicine. *Antioxidants & Redox Signaling, 27*(10), 684–712.

Cronin, O., Barton, W., Skuse, P., Penney, N. C., Garcia-Perez, I., Murphy, E. F., ... Falvey, E. C. (2018). A prospective metagenomic and metabolomic analysis of the impact of exercise and/or whey protein supplementation on the gut microbiome of sedentary adults. *mSystems, 3*(3), e00044-18.

Cui, X., Ye, L., Li, J., Jin, L., Wang, W., Li, S., ... Zhou, X. (2018). Metagenomic and metabolomic analyses unveil dysbiosis of gut microbiota in chronic heart failure patients. *Scientific Reports*, *8*(1), 635.

Danhof, M. (2016). Systems pharmacology–towards the modeling of network interactions. *European Journal of Pharmaceutical Sciences*, *94*, 4–14.

Derbal, Y. (2018). The adaptive complexity of cancer. *BioMed Research International*, *2018*.

Docci, L., Parrott, N., Krähenbühl, S., & Fowler, S. (2019). Application of new cellular and microphysiological systems to drug metabolism optimization and their positioning respective to in silico tools. *SLAS Discovery: Advancing Life Sciences R & D*, *24*, 523–536.

Doerr, S., Harvey, M. J., Noé, F., & De Fabritiis, G. (2016). HTMD: High-throughput molecular dynamics for molecular discovery. *Journal of Chemical Theory and Computation*, *12*(4), 1845–1852.

Dorrestein, P. C., Mazmanian, S. K., & Knight, R. (2014). Finding the missing links among metabolites, microbes, and the host. *Immunity*, *40*(6), 824–832.

Egorova, K. S., Gordeev, E. G., & Ananikov, V. P. (2017). Biological activity of ionic liquids and their application in pharmaceutics and medicine. *Chemical Reviews*, *117*(10), 7132–7189.

Farnsworth, K. (2018). How organisms gained causal independence and how it might be quantified. *Biology*, 7(3), 38.

Gacek, A., & Strauss, J. (2012). The chromatin code of fungal secondary metabolite gene clusters. *Applied Microbiology and Biotechnology*, *95*(6), 1389–1404.

Geschwindner, S., Ulander, J., & Johansson, P. (2015). Ligand binding thermodynamics in drug discovery: Still a hot tip? *Journal of Medicinal Chemistry*, *58*(16), 6321–6335.

Gogna, N., Sharma, R., Gupta, V., Dorai, K., & Prasad, N. G. (2017). Evolution of the metabolome in response to selection for increased immunity in populations of *Drosophila melanogaster*. *PLoS One*, *12*(11), e0188089.

Gohlke, A., Bower, J., Brown, P. N., Cameron, K. S., Drysdale, M., Goodwin, G., ... Mezna, M. (2018). A central role for biophysics in cancer drug discovery-development of candidate small molecule inhibitors in mutant KRas. *Biophysical Journal*, *114*(3), 30a–31a.

Guerriero, G., Berni, R., Muñoz-Sanchez, J., Apone, F., Abdel-Salam, E., Qahtan, A., ... Siddiqui, K. (2018). Production of plant secondary metabolites: Examples, tips and suggestions for biotechnologists. *Genes*, *9*(6), 309.

Haddad, W. (2017). Thermodynamics: The unique universal science. *Entropy*, *19*(11), 621.

Hallmann, A. (2015). Algae biotechnology–green cell-factories on the rise. *Current Biotechnology*, *4*(4), 389–415.

Hartung, T., FitzGerald, R. E., Jennings, P., Mirams, G. R., Peitsch, M. C., Rostami-Hodjegan, A., ... Sturla, S. J. (2017). Systems toxicology: Real world applications and opportunities. *Chemical Research in Toxicology*, *30*(4), 870–882.

Hasson, S. A., & Inglese, J. (2013). Innovation in academic chemical screening: Filling the gaps in chemical biology. *Current Opinion in Chemical Biology*, *17*(3), 329–338.

Hoelder, S., Clarke, P. A., & Workman, P. (2012). Discovery of small molecule cancer drugs: Successes, challenges and opportunities. *Molecular Oncology*, *6*(2), 155–176.

Holdgate, G., Geschwindner, S., Breeze, A., Davies, G., Colclough, N., Temesi, D., & Ward, L. (2013). Biophysical methods in drug discovery from small molecule to pharmaceutical. *Methods in Molecular Biology (Clifton, NJ)*, *1008*, 327.

Ildefonso, M. (2015). Elements of the cellular metabolic structure. *Frontiers in Molecular Biosciences*, *2*.

Ingber, D. (2018). Biophysics-enabled translational medicine. *Biophysical Journal*, *114*(3), 23a.

Jain, K. K. (2013). Synthetic biology and personalized medicine. *Medical Principles and Practice*, *22*(3), 209–219.

Johnson, C. H., Ivanisevic, J., & Siuzdak, G. (2016). Metabolomics: Beyond biomarkers and towards mechanisms. *Nature Reviews Molecular Cell Biology*, *17*(7), 451.

Joslin, J., Gilligan, J., Anderson, P., Garcia, C., Sharif, O., Hampton, J., … Trussell, C. (2018). A fully automated high-throughput flow cytometry screening system enabling phenotypic drug discovery. *SLAS Discovery: Advancing Life Sciences R&D*, *23*(7), 697–707.

Juster, R. P., Russell, J. J., Almeida, D., & Picard, M. (2016). Allostatic load and comorbidities: A mitochondrial, epigenetic, and evolutionary perspective. *Development and Psychopathology*, *28*(4Pt1), 1117–1146.

Kakaç, S., Kosoy, B., Li, D., & Pramuanjaroenkij, A. (Eds.), (2010). *Microfluidics based microsystems: Fundamentals and applications*. Springer.

Katz, L., Chen, Y.Y., Gonzalez, R., Peterson, T. C., Zhao, H., & Baltz, R. H. (2018). Synthetic biology advances and applications in the biotechnology industry: A perspective. *Journal of Industrial Microbiology & Biotechnology*, *45*(7), 449–461.

Kell, D. B. (2013). Finding novel pharmaceuticals in the systems biology era using multiple effective drug targets, phenotypic screening and knowledge of transporters: Where drug discovery went wrong and how to fix it. *The FEBS Journal*, *280*(23), 5957–5980.

Klassen, A., Faccio, A. T., Canuto, G. A., da Cruz, P. L., Ribeiro, H. C., Tavares, M. F., & Sussulini, A. (2017). Metabolomics: Definitions and significance in systems biology. *Advances in Experimental Medicine and Biology*, *965*, 3.

Koskella, B., Hall, L. J., & Metcalf, C. J. E. (2017). The microbiome beyond the horizon of ecological and evolutionary theory. *Nature Ecology & Evolution*, *1*(11), 1606.

Kumar, R. R., & Prasad, S. (2011). Metabolic engineering of bacteria. *Indian Journal of Microbiology*, *51*(3), 403–409.

Le Feuvre, R. A., & Scrutton, N. S. (2018). A living foundry for synthetic biological materials: A synthetic biology roadmap to new advanced materials. *Synthetic and Systems Biotechnology*, *3*(2), 105–112.

Liang, Y., & Kelemen, A. (2017). Computational dynamic approaches for temporal omics data with applications to systems medicine. *BioData Mining*, *10*(1), 20.

Ma, X., & Zhao, Y. (2014). Biomedical applications of supramolecular systems based on host–guest interactions. *Chemical Reviews*, *115*(15), 7794–7839.

Madani Tonekaboni, S. A., Soltan Ghoraie, L., Manem, V. S. K., & Haibe-Kains, B. (2016). Predictive approaches for drug combination discovery in cancer. *Briefings in Bioinformatics*, *19*(2), 263–276.

Maley, C. C., Aktipis, A., Graham, T. A., Sottoriva, A., Boddy, A. M., Janiszewska, M., … Anderson, K. S. (2017). Classifying the evolutionary and ecological features of neoplasms. *Nature Reviews Cancer*, *17*(10), 605.

Mao, L., & Franke, J. (2015). Symbiosis, dysbiosis, and rebiosis—The value of metaproteomics in human microbiome monitoring. *Proteomics*, *15*(5–6), 1142–1151.

Markley, J. L., Brüschweiler, R., Edison, A. S., Eghbalnia, H. R., Powers, R., Raftery, D., & Wishart, D. S. (2017). The future of NMR-based metabolomics. *Current Opinion in Biotechnology*, *43*, 34–40.

Martinez Molina, D., & Nordlund, P. (2016). The cellular thermal shift assay: A novel biophysical assay for in situ drug target engagement and mechanistic biomarker studies. *Annual Review of Pharmacology and Toxicology*, *56*, 141–161.

Marx, U., Andersson, T. B., Bahinski, A., Beilmann, M., Beken, S., Cassee, F. R., … Gaertner, C. (2016). Biology-inspired microphysiological system approaches to solve the prediction dilemma of substance testing. *ALTEX*, *33*(3), 272.

Metallo, C. M., & Vander Heiden, M. G. (2013). Understanding metabolic regulation and its influence on cell physiology. *Molecular Cell*, *49*(3), 388–398.

Milani, C., Duranti, S., Bottacini, F., Casey, E., Turroni, F., Mahony, J., … Lugli, G. A. (2017). The first microbial colonizers of the human gut: Composition, activities, and health implications of the infant gut microbiota. *Microbiology and Molecular Biology Reviews*, *81*(4), e00036-17.

Miller, J. V., Prince, N., Mouch, J. A., & Boyd, J. W. (2019). *A toxicological application of signal transduction: Early cellular changes can be indicative of toxicity*. In *Cellular signal transduction in toxicology and pharmacology: Data collection, analysis, and interpretation*. Hoboken, NJ: John Wiley & Sons. (pp. 239–266).

Mirsadeghi, S., & Larijani, B. (2017). Personalized medicine: Pharmacogenomics and drug development. *Acta Medica Iranica*, 150–165.

Möller, C., & Slack, M. (2010). Impact of new technologies for cellular screening along the drug value chain. *Drug Discovery Today*, *15*(9–10), 384–390.

Mori, Y., & Shirai, T. (2018). Designing artificial metabolic pathways, construction of target enzymes, and analysis of their function. *Current Opinion in Biotechnology*, *54*, 41–44.

Nikolaev, E. V. (2010). The elucidation of metabolic pathways and their improvements using stable optimization of large-scale kinetic models of cellular systems. *Metabolic Engineering*, *12*(1), 26–38.

Nussinov, R., Jang, H., Tsai, C. J., & Cheng, F. (2019). Precision medicine review: Rare driver mutations and their biophysical classification. *Biophysical Reviews*, *11*(1), 5–19.

Ouldridge, T. E. (2018). The importance of thermodynamics for molecular systems, and the importance of molecular systems for thermodynamics. *Natural Computing*, *17*(1), 3–29.

Peng, B., Li, H., & Peng, X. X. (2015). Functional metabolomics: From biomarker discovery to metabolome reprogramming. *Protein & Cell*, *6*(9), 628–637.

Pickens, L. B., Tang, Y., & Chooi, Y. H. (2011). Metabolic engineering for the production of natural products. *Annual Review of Chemical and Biomolecular Engineering*, *2*, 211–236.

Pimenta, L. P., Kim, H. K., Verpoorte, R., & Choi, Y. H. (2013). NMR-based metabolomics: A probe to utilize biodiversity. *Methods in Molecular Biology (Clifton, NJ)*, *1055*, 117.

Porcar, M. (2019). The hidden charm of life. *Life*, *9*(1), 5.

Postler, T. S., & Ghosh, S. (2017). Understanding the holobiont: How microbial metabolites affect human health and shape the immune system. *Cell Metabolism*, *26*(1), 110–130.

Preidis, G. A., & Hotez, P. J. (2015). The newest "omics"—Metagenomics and metabolomics—Enter the battle against the neglected tropical diseases. *PLoS Neglected Tropical Diseases*, *9*(2), e0003382.

Prosser, G. A., Larrouy-Maumus, G., & de Carvalho, L. P. S. (2014). Metabolomic strategies for the identification of new enzyme functions and metabolic pathways. *EMBO Reports*, *15*(6), 657–669.

Rai, A., Saito, K., & Yamazaki, M. (2017). Integrated omics analysis of specialized metabolism in medicinal plants. *The Plant Journal*, *90*(4), 764–787.

Ramsay, R. R., Popovic-Nikolic, M. R., Nikolic, K., Uliassi, E., & Bolognesi, M. L. (2018). A perspective on multi-target drug discovery and design for complex diseases. *Clinical and Translational Medicine*, 7(1), 3.

Renaud, J. P., Chung, C. W., Danielson, U. H., Egner, U., Hennig, M., Hubbard, R. E., & Nar, H. (2016). Biophysics in drug discovery: Impact, challenges and opportunities. *Nature Reviews Drug Discovery*, *15*(10), 679.

Renda, B. A., Hammerling, M. J., & Barrick, J. E. (2014). Engineering reduced evolutionary potential for synthetic biology. *Molecular BioSystems*, *10*(7), 1668–1678.

Richier, S., Furla, P., Plantivaux, A., Merle, P. L., & Allemand, D. (2005). Symbiosis-induced adaptation to oxidative stress. *Journal of Experimental Biology*, *208*(2), 277–285.

Rook, G., Bäckhed, F., Levin, B. R., McFall-Ngai, M. J., & McLean, A. R. (2017). Evolution, human-microbe interactions, and life history plasticity. *The Lancet*, *390*(10093), 521–530.

Rooks, M. G., & Garrett, W. S. (2016). Gut microbiota, metabolites and host immunity. *Nature Reviews Immunology*, *16*(6), 341.

Rosato, A., Tenori, L., Cascante, M., Carulla, P.R.D.A., dos Santos, V. A. M., & Saccenti, E. (2018). From correlation to causation: Analysis of metabolomics data using systems biology approaches. *Metabolomics*, *14*(4), 37.

Rosenberg, E., & Zilber-Rosenberg, I. (2011). Symbiosis and development: The hologenome concept. *Birth Defects Research Part C: Embryo Today: Reviews*, *93*(1), 56–66.
Rosenberg, E., & Zilber-Rosenberg, I. (2018). The hologenome concept of evolution after 10 years. *Microbiome*, *6*(1), 78.
Rosenberg, E., & Zilber-Rosenberg, I. (2019). The hologenome concept of evolution: Medical implications. *Rambam Maimonides Medical Journal*, *10*(1).
Saltepe, B., Kehribar, E. S., Su Yirmibeşoğlu, S. S., & Şafak Şeker, U. O. (2017). Cellular biosensors with engineered genetic circuits. *ACS Sensors*, *3*(1), 13–26.
Sánchez-Rodríguez, A., Pérez-Castillo, Y., Schürer, S. C., Nicolotti, O., Mangiatordi, G. F., Borges, F., … Cruz-Monteagudo, M. (2017). From flamingo dance to (desirable) drug discovery: A nature-inspired approach. *Drug Discovery Today*, *22*(10), 1489–1502.
Schmidt-Dannert, C., & Lopez-Gallego, F. (2016). A roadmap for biocatalysis–functional and spatial orchestration of enzyme cascades. *Microbial Biotechnology*, *9*(5), 601–609.
Schuetz, D. A., de Witte, W. E. A., Wong, Y. C., Knasmueller, B., Richter, L., Kokh, D. B., … Segala, E. (2017). Kinetics for drug discovery: An industry-driven effort to target drug residence time. *Drug Discovery Today*, *22*(6), 896–911.
Scott, T. A., Quintaneiro, L. M., Norvaisas, P., Lui, P. P., Wilson, M. P., Leung, K.Y., … Bryson, K. (2017). Host-microbe co-metabolism dictates cancer drug efficacy in *C. elegans*. *Cell*, *169*(3), 442–456.
Selber-Hnatiw, S., Rukundo, B., Ahmadi, M., Akoubi, H., Al-Bizri, H., Aliu, A. F., … Begum, F. (2017). Human gut microbiota: Toward an ecology of disease. *Frontiers in Microbiology*, *8*, 1265.
Selvarajoo, K. (2015). Can the second law of thermodynamics hold in cell cultures? *Frontiers in Genetics*, *6*, 262.
Sengupta, B., Stemmler, M. B., & Friston, K. J. (2013). Information and efficiency in the nervous system—A synthesis. *PLoS Computational Biology*, *9*(7), e1003157.
Shapira, M. (2016). Gut microbiotas and host evolution: Scaling up symbiosis. *Trends in Ecology & Evolution*, *31*(7), 539–549.
Shapiro, J. (2017). Living organisms author their read-write genomes in evolution. *Biology*, *6*(4), 42.
Sharma, A. K., Jaiswal, S. K., Chaudhary, N., & Sharma, V. K. (2017). A novel approach for the prediction of species-specific biotransformation of xenobiotic/drug molecules by the human gut microbiota. *Scientific Reports*, 7(1), 9751.
Shi-Kai, Y., Run-Hui, L., Hui-Zi, J., Xin-Ru, L., Ji, Y., Lei, S., & Zhang, W. D. (2015). "Omics" in pharmaceutical research: Overview, applications, challenges, and future perspectives. *Chinese Journal of Natural Medicines*, *13*(1), 3–21.
Shimada, I., Ueda, T., Kofuku, Y., Eddy, M. T., & Wüthrich, K. (2018). GPCR drug discovery: Integrating solution NMR data with crystal and cryo-EM structures. *Nature Reviews Drug Discovery*, *18*(1), 59–82.
Singh, S. B., & Pelaez, F. (2008). *Biodiversity, chemical diversity and drug discovery*. In Vol. I. *Natural compounds as drugs*. Basel: Birkhäuser. (pp. 141–174).
Smanski, M. J., Zhou, H., Claesen, J., Shen, B., Fischbach, M. A., & Voigt, C. A. (2016). Synthetic biology to access and expand nature's chemical diversity. *Nature Reviews Microbiology*, *14*(3), 135.
Smith, R. W., van Sluijs, B., & Fleck, C. (2017). Designing synthetic networks in silico: A generalised evolutionary algorithm approach. *BMC Systems Biology*, *11*(1), 118.
Stano, P. (2019). Is research on "synthetic cells" moving to the next level? *Life*, *9*(1), 3.
Stern, A. M., Schurdak, M. E., Bahar, I., Berg, J. M., & Taylor, D. L. (2016). A perspective on implementing a quantitative systems pharmacology platform for drug discovery and the advancement of personalized medicine. *Journal of Biomolecular Screening*, *21*(6), 521–534.
Tebani, A., & Bekri, S. (2019). Paving the way to precision nutrition through metabolomics. *Frontiers in Nutrition*, *6*.

Thomas, S., Izard, J., Walsh, E., Batich, K., Chongsathidkiet, P., Clarke, G., … Gilligan, J. P. (2017). The host microbiome regulates and maintains human health: A primer and perspective for non-microbiologists. *Cancer Research*, 77(8), 1783–1812.

Tolstikov, V. (2016). Metabolomics: Bridging the gap between pharmaceutical development and population health. *Metabolites*, *6*(3), 20.

Tóth, A., Brózik, A., Szakács, G., Sarkadi, B., & Hegedüs, T. (2015). A novel mathematical model describing adaptive cellular drug metabolism and toxicity in the chemoimmune system. *PLoS One*, *10*(2), e0115533.

Trosset, J. Y., & Carbonell, P. (2015). Synthetic biology for pharmaceutical drug discovery. *Drug Design, Development and Therapy*, *9*, 6285.

Turnbaugh, P. J., & Gordon, J. I. (2008). An invitation to the marriage of metagenomics and metabolomics. *Cell*, *134*(5), 708–713.

Vaiserman, A. M. (2011). Hormesis and epigenetics: Is there a link? *Ageing Research Reviews*, *10*(4), 413–421.

Vangala, S., Pinjari, J., Patole, P., Ravindran, S., Gangal, R., Wangikar, P., … Rastogi, H. (2011). *Translational drug discovery research: Integration of medicinal chemistry, computational modeling, pharmacology, ADME, and toxicology*. In *Encyclopedia of drug metabolism and interactions*. Hoboken, NJ: John Wiley & Sons. (pp. 1–54).

Vernocchi, P., Vannini, L., Gottardi, D., Del Chierico, F., Serrazanetti, D. I., Ndagijimana, M., & Guerzoni, M. E. (2012). Integration of datasets from different analytical techniques to assess the impact of nutrition on human metabolome. *Frontiers in Cellular and Infection Microbiology*, *2*, 156.

Wei, Z., Xi, J., Gao, S., You, X., Li, N., Cao, Y., … Dong, X. (2018). Metabolomics coupled with pathway analysis characterizes metabolic changes in response to BDE-3 induced reproductive toxicity in mice. *Scientific Reports*, *8*(1), 5423.

Wen, H., Jung, H., & Li, X. (2015). Drug delivery approaches in addressing clinical pharmacology-related issues: Opportunities and challenges. *The AAPS Journal*, *17*(6), 1327–1340.

Wishart, D. S. (2016). Emerging applications of metabolomics in drug discovery and precision medicine. *Nature Reviews Drug Discovery*, *15*(7), 473.

Yang, H., Sun, L., Wang, Z., Li, W., Liu, G., & Tang, Y. (2018). ADMETopt: A web server for ADMET optimization in drug design via scaffold hopping. *Journal of Chemical Information and Modeling*, *58*(10), 2051–2056.

Zahrl, R. J., Peña, D. A., Mattanovich, D., & Gasser, B. (2017). Systems biotechnology for protein production in *Pichia pastoris*. *FEMS Yeast Research*, *17*(7), fox068.

Zakrewsky, M., Lovejoy, K. S., Kern, T. L., Miller, T. E., Le, V., Nagy, A., … Fox, D. T. (2014). Ionic liquids as a class of materials for transdermal delivery and pathogen neutralization. *Proceedings of the National Academy of Sciences*, *111*(37), 13313–13318.

Zhao, L., Nicholson, J. K., Lu, A., Wang, Z., Tang, H., Holmes, E., … Lindon, J. C. (2012). Targeting the human genome–microbiome axis for drug discovery: Inspirations from global systems biology and traditional Chinese medicine. *Journal of Proteome Research*, *11*(7), 3509–3519.

Zivieri, R., Pacini, N., Finocchio, G., & Carpentieri, M. (2017). Rate of entropy model for irreversible processes in living systems. *Scientific Reports*, 7(1), 9134.

Zou, J., Zheng, M. W., Li, G., & Su, Z. G. (2013). Advanced systems biology methods in drug discovery and translational biomedicine. *BioMed Research International*, *2013*.

Index

Note: Page numbers followed by *f* indicate figures.

F

G

H

I

J

L

M

Kolibri 360 GmbH
Ferdinand-Jühlke-Straße 7
99095 Erfurt, Deutschland
produktsicherheit@kolibri360.de